Dr. Homola's
Macro-Nutrient Diet
for Quick, Permanent
Weight Loss

Books by Samuel Homola

Bonesetting, Chiropractic, and Cultism

Backache: Home Treatment and Prevention

Muscle Training for Athletes

A Chiropractor's Treasury of Health Secrets

Secrets of Naturally Youthful Health and Vitality

Doctor Homola's Natural Health Remedies

Doctor Homola's Life-Extender Health Guide

Doctor Homola's Fat-Disintegrator Diet

Peter Lupus' Guide to Radiant Health and Beauty: Mission Possible for Women (with Peter Lupus)

Peter Lupus' Celebrity Body Book: A Body-Improvement Guide for Men and Women (with Peter Lupus)

Dr. Homola's Macro-Nutrient Diet for Quick, Permanent Weight Loss

SAMUEL HOMOLA, D.C.

Parker Publishing Company, Inc.   West Nyack, N.Y.

Library of Congress Cataloging in Publication Data

Homola, Samuel.
    Dr. Homola's macro-nutrient diet for quick
permanent weight loss.

    Includes index.
    1. Reducing diets.   2. High-fiber diet—Recipes.
3. Food, Natural.   I. Title.   II. Title: Macro-
nutrient diet for quick permanent weight loss.
RM222.2.H586   613.2'5   81-38340
ISBN 0-13-216952-5   AACR2

Dedicated to my wife, Martha,

and to her two most helpful friends,

Helen Ingram and Margie Smith.

FOREWORD BY A DOCTOR OF MEDICINE

The science of nutrition has made tremendous advances in recent years. These advances have not always been evident in some popular reducing diets, however. As a practicing physician, I am more concerned than ever about the proliferation of bad reducing diets. Ignoring all the rules of good nutrition, many fad diets restrict consumption of such important foods as fruits and vegetables. Low-carbohydrate diets, for example, produce dramatic but dangerous weight loss by draining water from the body. Some high-fat diets endanger health by contributing to the development of cancer, atherosclerosis, and other diseases.

There is, at present, a great deal of controversy surrounding the use of diet in the treatment and prevention of disease. The science of nutrition is not yet complete. All of the answers are not yet known when it comes to the role of diet in the development of disease. So there is room for differences in opinion. Some bad reducing diets, however, ignore the fundamentals of good dieting. The basic food groups, for example, are just as important today as they were when they were first developed. Elimination of any basic food group without good medical reasons is likely to result in a bad diet that contributes to the development of disease.

Dietary Goals for the United States, published by the U.S. Senate in 1977, provides a sensible guide for Americans seeking dietary information. Using the U.S. Senate publication as a reference, Dr. Homola has developed a safe, sensible reducing diet for Americans who are concerned about their health. Combining common sense with basic science, his diet will benefit all who follow it.

This new book by Dr. Homola will clear up any confusion you have about dieting. You'll be able to use it to control your weight and protect your health for years to come. I recommend it highly. I predict that Dr. Homola's book will be read by millions of people who are seeking better health and a slimmer body.

Joseph L. Kaplowe, M.D.

7

What This Book Is All About— and What It Can Do for You

"I've been on every diet known to man," complained comedian Paul Lynde, "and I succeeded on all of them. But the weight always comes back. Someone should write a book on how to keep the weight off when you lose it."

Here, at last, is a book describing a *permanent* weight-loss diet that will trim excess body fat and keep it off. This new dieting method is based on the new U.S. Dietary Goals—and it is not a fad diet. Instead, it is a sensible diet that assures good health as well as permanent weight loss.

A DIET FOR EVERYONE

Overweight is a common problem in America. It has been estimated that one of every three Americans is overweight. About 20 percent of all adults are obese. "Obesity is probably the most common and one of the most serious nutritional problems affecting the American public today," said a U.S. Senate Select Committee studying nutrition in America.

Obesity can be a factor in the development of cardiovascular disease, high blood pressure, atherosclerosis, hernia, gallbladder disease, diabetes mellitus, and liver disease. Too much body fat places an extra burden on the spine, hips, knees, and feet. Abdominal muscles often stretch, resulting in hernia. Fat stored in the abdomen literally pushes the stomach up through the diaphragm, encroaching upon the heart and lungs. Breathing is difficult and

9

circulation poor. The body as a whole performs poorly and becomes repulsive in appearance.

Even if you aren't obese, bad eating habits can contribute to the development of disease. According to *Dietary Goals for the United States,** six of the 10 leading causes of death in the United States are linked to our diet. Foods deficient in fiber and nutrients and rich in saturated fat, salt, sugar, and cholesterol contribute to the development of heart disease, diabetes, cancer, stroke, and other killer diseases. Breast cancer and heart disease, for example, have been linked to a high-fat diet. Evidence indicates that colon cancer can be caused by dietary fat as well as by lack of adequate fiber in diets made up primarily of processed foods. Increased consumption of sugar is believed to be responsible for the increasing incidence of diabetes. Hypertension (high blood pressure) may be triggered by overconsumption of salt, and so on.

Because of the way we eat, one of every three men in the United States can be expected to die of heart disease or stroke before the age of 60! Cancer is already the second leading cause of death in America. Diabetes is in seventh place and rising rapidly. More than 5,000,000 Americans now suffer from diabetes.

EATING TO PREVENT DISEASE

Good eating habits can *prevent* many diseases as well as reduce excess body fat. Unfortunately, most reducing diets are concerned only with loss of body weight as quickly as possible—and this usually means a *bad* diet that contributes to the development of disease. Many low-calorie diets, for example, are deficient in essential nutrients. High-protein and high-fat diets are loaded with saturated fat and cholesterol, and they are deficient in fiber. Low-carbohydrate diets are deficient in nutrients as well as fiber.

The trend in fad diets in recent years has been to drastically reduce carbohydrate intake and increase consumption of protein and fat. Today, most Americans get only a little more than 20 percent of their calories from such natural fiber-rich carbohydrates as fresh fruits, vegetables, and whole grains. Sugar and refined carbohydrates supply about 24 percent of calories, with about 42

*Superintendent of Documents, U.S. Government Printing Office, Washington, D.C. 20402, December, 1977.

percent of calories coming from fat. This means that the average American's diet is low in fiber and natural carbohydrates and high in sugar and fat. You don't have to be a doctor to see the dangers of such a diet.

THE ANSWER: THE NEW MACRO-NUTRIENT DIET

We now know that *natural carbohydrates* are the best and the cleanest source of energy for the body. There is also evidence to indicate that natural carbohydrates are much less fattening than protein and fat. One reason for this is that natural carbohydrate foods are rich in water and fiber and therefore provide more bulk with fewer calories. The authors of *Dietary Goals* have informed us that ". . . an increase in the consumption of complex carbohydrates is likely to erase the problem of weight control." And they add that a diet high in complex (natural) carbohydrate will reduce the risk of heart disease, diabetes, and other diseases by displacing sugar and fat in the diet.

So, in the interest of disease prevention as well as weight control, the new U.S. Dietary Goals recommend that Americans *increase* their consumption of natural carbohydrate. This is the basis for my new macro-nutrient diet.

DIET CONTROL FOR SAFE WEIGHT LOSS

On a macro-nutrient diet, you'll learn how to use calorie control as a *reducing power pedal* for slow or fast weight loss. You'll be able to adjust your *fat-burner throttle* by manipulating the macro-nutrients in your diet so that carbohydrate, protein, and fat are kept in correct proportions. When your weight has been reduced to a desirable level, you can ease up on your power pedal and pull back on your throttle a little. You'll be able to *increase* your intake of delicious natural carbohydrate foods so that they supply up to 58 percent of your total intake of calories.

A NEW, DIFFERENT DIET

My new macro-nutrient diet is completely different from the dangerous high-fat, high-protein, and low-carbohydrate diets that are now so popular. A slimming diet and a maintenance diet based on the new U.S. Dietary Goals will improve your health and lengthen your life as well as rid your body of excess fat. This same dietary approach will *prevent* some of the diseases that are common causes of death.

If there ever is a "diet revolution," it will take place with the realization that *natural fiber-rich carbohydrates are the most healthful and the least fattening of all the foods.* The diet outlined in this book will project you into the future, providing you with all the benefits of good nutrition. Armed with the knowledge of how to control and balance your intake of calories and macro-nutrients with sensible, lifetime eating habits, you can forever avoid the use of fad diets that provide temporary weight loss at the expense of your health.

The new macro-nutrient diet is low in fat, salt, sugar, and cholesterol—and it's high in fiber, water, and nutrients. It's everything you'll ever need for building and maintaining good health and a slim body.

Samuel Homola, D.C.

CONTENTS

Foreword by a Doctor of Medicine 7

What This Book Is All About—and What It Can Do For You 9

1 Solve Your Weight Problem with Special, Nutritious
   Macro-Nutrient Foods 17

   You Must Change Your Eating Habits • 18
   Why a Macro-Nutrient Diet Is Superior to other Diets • 19
   How to Avoid Dangerous Diet Revolutions • 20
   The Case for Carbohydrates • 22
   The U.S. Dietary Goals • 25
   Eat and Enjoy on a Macro-Nutrient Diet! • 28
   The Seven Basic Food Groups • 29
   The Basic Four Food Groups • 30
   General Rules for Healthful Eating on a Slimming Diet • 30
   A Sample Natural-Food Diet Plan • 35
   Taking the Ignorance out of Dieting • 36
   Summary • 38

2 How to Adjust Your Fat-Burner Throttle on an Effortless Slimming
   Program with Macro-Nutrient Foods 39

   How to Adjust Energy Nutrients on a 1,200 Calorie Diet • 40
   How to Adjust Energy Nutrients on a 2,000 Calorie Diet • 40
   Patient, Long-Range Dieting Is Best • 42
   How to Develop a 1,200+ Calorie Diet • 44
   How to Calculate Energy-Nutrient Percentages • 46
   Sample Three-Meal Menu • 47
   You Are Unique • 48
   Keep Your Stomach Full with Macro-Nutrient Foods • 50
   Make Your Diet More Effective by Exercising • 51
   Summary • 52

3 **How to Control Your Reducing Power Pedal to Attain an Attractive, Ideal Body Weight with Macro-Nutrient Foods** **53**

How to Control Your Reducing Power Pedal by Tailoring Your
    Calorie Intake ● 54
How to Figure Calorie Requirement According to Body Weight ● 56
Weight Chart for Men ● 57
Weight Chart for Women ● 57
A Quick Review ● 59
Why Dieting Results Vary ● 61
Drink Plenty of Water and Reduce Your Salt Intake ● 63
What About Fasting ? ● 66
Count Down on Body Fat ● 68
More Examples of Successful, Beneficial Weight Loss ● 70
Summary ● 71

4 **How to Get the Nutrients You Need from Delicious Macro-Nutrient Foods** **72**

Food Preparation Is Important ● 73
Adjusting to Food Problems ● 73
How to Get Your Share of Nutrients
    from the Milk Group ● 74
How to Get Meat Nutrients Without Fat ● 77
Balance Your Nutrient Intake with Vegetables
    and Fruits ● 81
The Special Nutrients of Whole-Grain Products ● 87
Keep Fats and Oils at a Minimum ● 90
Summary ● 93

5 **Special Macro-Nutrient Food Sources of Healthful, Low-Fat Protein .** **94**

Substituting Soybeans for Meat ● 96
Fish Supplies Fewer Calories Than Meat ● 99
How to Make Your Own Low-Fat Yogurt ● 101
Whole-Grain Homemade Bread Is Best! ● 102
Vegetarianism in a Reducing Diet ● 105
Complete Meal in a Salad ● 108
Health Drinks Substituted for Meals ● 109
Summary ● 113

6 How to Enrich Macro-Nutrient Foods for Safe, Rapid Weight Loss . 115

The Many Benefits of a High-Fiber Diet ● 116
Crude Fiber Content of Food Servings ● 125
Selecting and Preparing Fiber-Rich Foods ● 125
Summary ● 132

7 How to Nibble on Macro-Nutrient Foods for Pleasurable Slimming . 134

Four Methods of Nibbling ● 135
1. How to Eat Six Times a Day and Still
   Lose Weight ● 138
2. How to Kill Your Appetite by Nibbling
   on Raw Vegetables ● 141
3. How to Control Low Blood Sugar by
   Eating Between Meals ● 143
4. How to Kill Your Appetite with Zero-Calorie Fiber ● 146
Summary ● 148

8 Fun and Purpose in Eating Macro-Nutrient Foods Away from Home . 150

Restaurant Foods Are Often Low in Nutrients ● 150
Selecting Suitable Macro-Nutrient Foods
   When Dining Out ● 151
Tips from Celebrities on Eating Out ● 154
Variety in Your Lunch Box ● 157
Supplement Questionable Diets with Vitamins ● 159
Preventing Calcium and Iron Deficiencies ● 162
Everyone's Needs Are Different ● 164
Summary ● 165

9 The Lifetime Health-and-Body Benefits of Macro-Nutrient Foods . 166

A Reducing Diet That Builds Good Health! ● 166
Preventing Heart and Blood Vessel Disease
   with Macro-Nutrient Foods ● 169
How to Fight Cancer with a Macro-Nutrient Diet ● 173
Put a Stop to the Epidemic of Diabetes Mellitus ● 174
How to Adjust Your Diet to Relieve Gluten Allergy ● 175
How to Combat Diverticulitis with Fiber ● 176
How to Avoid Gouty Arthritis on a Reducing Diet ● 178
Fight Arthritis with Good Health and a Good Diet ● 179
Depending Upon the Wisdom of Your Body ● 181
Summary ● 182

10 Maintaining Good Health and an Ideal Body Weight with Macro-Nutrient Foods and a New Life Style **183**

You are Unique ● 184
Why You Should Include Exercise in Your
    Maintenance Program ● 184
How to Modify Your Behavior to Make Dieting Easier ● 189
Take Charge of Your Life ● 195
Summary ● 198

11 Everyday Macro-Nutrient Menus for Better Health and a Slimmer Body **199**

Pick the Diet Plan That Suits You Best ● 200
Follow This Three-Step Approach to a
    Macro-Nutrient Diet ● 200
The Special Benefits of a Macro-Nutrient Diet ● 202
A Rapid Weight-Loss 1,200+ Calorie Basic Diet Plan ● 204
Slower Weight Loss on a 1,500+ Calorie Diet Plan ● 206
Body Maintenance with a 2,500+ Calorie Diet Plan ● 207
Sample Basic Menus for Everyone ● 208
Use Common Sense and Imagination ● 212
Summary ● 213

12 Energy Nutrient Values of Common Carbohydrate, Protein, and Fat Macro-Nutrient Foods **214**

Report Your Results to Me ● 214
Table of Macro-Nutrient Values ● 215
Macro-Nutrient Food Sources of Important
    Micro-Nutrients ● 229

Index **231**

Solve Your Weight Problem
with Special, Nutritious
Macro-Nutrient Foods

There are many popular reducing diets that have proven to be effective in reducing body weight—at least temporarily. But not all of these diets are safe. Low-carbohydrate diets, for example, deprive the body of essential nutrients and create nutritional imbalances. Most popular fad diets are low in carbohydrate and high in protein and fat, and they generate many harmful by-products. Fats, in addition to being high in calories (nine calories per gram compared to four calories per gram of carbohydrate), form toxic ketones in the body when burned in the absence of carbohydrate.

An excessive amount of dietary fat is believed to contribute to the development of heart disease and cancer. Protein leaves a nitrogenous waste that must be eliminated by the kidneys. The purines in protein form uric acid in the body, resulting in gouty arthritis or kidney stones in susceptible persons. An excessive amount of protein or fat in a low-carbohydrate diet overworks the kidneys and dehydrates the body, resulting in a rapid, harmful, and temporary weight loss.

The February 28, 1980, issue of *The New England Journal of Medicine,* in comparing the effects of protein diets and mixed diets in reducing body weight, reported that a low-calorie protein diet results in excessive loss of sodium and water, a decrease in the function of the sympathetic nervous system, and an abnormal drop in blood pressure. It was also noted that a pure protein diet offers no protein-sparing advantage over a diet containing carbohydrate. "The increased losses of sodium and fluids could account entirely for the greater weight loss observed with the protein diet than with the mixed diet. . . . Low calorie protein diets thus cannot be viewed as more efficacious than mixed diets in the management of obesity and may, in fact, result in adverse effects not observed with carbohydrate-containing diets."

Dietary carbohydrate should, of course, be natural rather than refined. Natural carbohydrates are rich in water, fiber, vitamins, and minerals, providing filling, nutritious bulk with energy nutrients that burn clean with no toxic by-products. You can eat generous amounts of natural carbohydrates in a balanced diet. It's absolutely essential, however, to include some of *all* the basic energy nutrients—carbohydrate, protein, and fat—in a reducing diet for healthful, permanent weight loss. As you'll learn later in this chapter, a *high-carbohydrate* diet that includes some protein and fat is the best and the safest approach to take in dieting.

YOU MUST CHANGE YOUR EATING HABITS

Some fad diets that eliminate basic foods result in weight loss because they ultimately reduce calorie intake. Persons who eat only protein and fat, for example, simply do not eat as much as someone who has a greater variety of foods to choose from. But no one can follow such a restricted diet for very long. And when old eating habits are resumed, the lost weight quickly returns. If you want to get rid of excess body fat and keep it off, you'll have to change your eating habits and adopt a balanced diet that you can follow for the rest of your life. It's not enough to go on a short-term crash diet.

If you know how to diet, you can reduce your calorie intake by eating a variety of healthful foods in a balanced diet. You should never simplify dieting into such one-step procedures as eliminating carbohydrate or eating all the fat you want. Sensible dieting is not complicated. If you include generous amounts of natural carbohydrates in a balanced diet, as I recommend in my macro-nutrient diet, you'll be able to eat ample portions and still get rid of excess body fat. Best of all, your health will improve rather than deteriorate.

You Can Improve Your Life with a Macro-Nutrient Diet!

Angela P. suffered constantly from the physical discomfort and the mental embarrassment of carrying around excess body fat. Her self-confidence suffered, too. And all this resulted in problems for the whole family. Angela had quit attending school meetings on behalf of her children. Business and social functions were out of the question. Eating became the foremost pleasure in her life, so Angela continued to gain weight. She gained 68 pounds over a seven-year period, bringing her total body weight to an obese 218 pounds. "I can't go on like this," Angela lamented. "Life is becoming unbearable for me."

Fortunately, Angela stumbled upon the macro-nutrient principles of dieting and changed her eating habits. For the first time in her life, she learned enough about dieting to control her eating habits. *She lost 100 pounds in seven months.* At 118 pounds, she was transformed into a happy, beautiful, and confident woman. She began to participate in school activities with her children. Social functions became a pleasure rather than an embarrassment. "My whole life has been changed by my macro-nutrient diet," Angela stated emphatically. "Being 100 pounds lighter has improved my mental state as well as my physical appearance. This new dieting method has taught me how to eat for good health as well as how to eat for weight loss. And the foods I'm eating are really delicious! Best of all, I'm feeling so good that I'm now going after *all* the good things in life."

The last time I saw Angela, she was selling real estate, presiding over the local P.T.A., and taking disco lessons with her husband.

A macro-nutrient diet can change your life, too.

WHY A MACRO-NUTRIENT DIET IS SUPERIOR TO OTHER DIETS

You don't have to lose a hundred pounds to experience the benefits of a macro-nutrient diet. Even if you have only a few pounds to lose, or if you have no excess body fat at all, you can use a macro-nutrient diet to improve your health and prolong your life. So whether you're obese, only moderately overweight, or slim and trim, you will experience healthful benefits on a macro-nutrient diet. *This new method of dieting offers more health benefits than any other method of dieting.* For the first time, you'll be able to manipulate your diet for truly *healthful* weight loss. With this new, different dieting approach, you'll develop a slimmer, healthier body that will contribute to a better life. And you'll be able to look forward to a lifetime of eating delicious, healthful foods.

Special Benefits of a Macro-Nutrient Diet

Theola K. had to lose 58 pounds to prepare for gallbladder surgery. She accomplished this quite easily in eight months on a macro-nutrient diet. Without the excess abdominal fat, surgery was simple and uncomplicated and healing was rapid. But there were some additional benefits. Theola's physical appearance improved so much that she purchased new clothes, took a charm course, and landed a job as a hostess in an exclusive restaurant.

The course of Theola's life was drastically altered for the better as a result of shedding ugly fat on a macro-nutrient diet. "I hate to think where I'd be and what I'd look like today if I had not been forced to begin eating sensibly," Theola reflected with a shudder. "My macro-nutrient diet has truly worked wonders in my life."

Colline T. had only 25 pounds to lose, and it took her six months to lose it. But at her new weight of 123 pounds, she experienced a renewed interest in life. "Simply looking better makes you feel better," Colline insists. "And when you look better and feel better, everything in life is better—and I mean *everything!*"

Your macro-nutrient diet will produce many unexpected benefits. In addition to discovering new taste treats, you can expect to see and feel many changes for the better in yourself when you go on a macro-nutrient diet. If you follow the instructions outlined in this book, I promise that you'll be able to lose weight healthfully and permanently on a generous diet of delicious, natural foods. And I guarantee that you'll feel better than you have ever felt before.

Once you have tried the macro-nutrient method of dieting, you won't be tempted to try a dangerous fad diet.

HOW TO AVOID DANGEROUS DIET REVOLUTIONS

When the "diet revolution" started with high-fat, zero-carbohydrate diets, many dieters thought their prayers had been answered. All they had to do to lose weight was to eliminate carbo-hydrates and eat all the protein and fat they wanted. As on other low-carbohydrate diets, weight loss was rapid because of excessive loss of body water. Forced burning of only fat and protein for energy loaded the blood with ketones and uric acid, resulting in foul breath, frequent urination, fatigue, depression, low blood pressure, inflamed joints, and other undesirable side effects. Loss of more than one pound of body weight a day resulted in serious dehydration. Large amounts of saturated fat and cholesterol in the blood threatened the heart and blood vessels. When the diet was discontinued and consumption of carbohydrates resumed, the body quickly regained lost water and body weight increased rapidly. In many cases, the body was permanently damaged. Pre-dictably, the popularity of the high-fat diet soon faded.

But American dieters had not yet learned their lesson. When the liquid protein diet arrived on the scene, it guaranteed weight loss when everything else had failed. Like other fad diets, it simplified dieting into a one-step procedure: substituting liquid protein for meals. Actor Ed Asner tried the liquid protein diet and found that he had to supplement the diet with fish and salads. "I believe I could have skipped the liquid protein and gotten better results," he observed.

Actually, liquid protein was a poor substitute for the real thing. Made from the hides and horns of animals, liquid protein was incomplete and had to be processed and supplemented with amino acids. The idea was to provide enough supplementary pro-tein to prevent the body from feeding on its muscles while burning stored fat. But without carbohydrate, fasting with liquid protein proved to be one of the most dangerous diets ever. Body metabolism was disturbed. Blood levels of essential vitamins and minerals dropped while ketones, uric acid, and other harmful products increased. Overloaded kidneys excreted water, calcium, sodium, potassium, and other nutrients that were essential for the function of the heart and other organs. Serious dehydration re-sulted. When potassium got too low, the heart stopped beating. It has been estimated that as many as 58 persons may have died as a result of going on a liquid protein diet! (*Diets '79*, Consumer Guide.)

Meeting Minimum Dietary Requirements

When you go on a diet that is not medically supervised, it's important to make sure that you supply your body with *at least* 100 grams of carbohydrate, 60 grams of protein, and 1,200 calories. You may take in considerably more carbohydrate on a reducing diet if foods are selected carefully. And to make sure that you supply your body with adequate vitamins and minerals, you *must* select something from each of the basic food groups each day. You must have a certain amount of carbohydrate in your diet to burn fat adequately. Carbohydrate also reduces protein requirement, but you must have all three energy nutrients—carbohydrate, protein, and fat—in your diet for good health. There is no satisfactory substitute for the balanced diet approach in building good health or reducing body weight.

THE CASE FOR CARBOHYDRATES

In the early 1900's, about 40 percent of our calorie intake came from such fiber-rich natural carbohydrates as fresh fruits, vegetables, and whole-grain cereals. In those days, obesity was not so common. Today, only about 20 percent of the average American's daily calorie intake comes from natural carbohydrates. Fiber-rich carbohydrates have been replaced by fat-rich meats such as beef and pork and by refined carbohydrates which are often enriched with sugar, salt, and fat. As a result, the incidence of obesity and associated killer diseases has risen dramatically. Because of this, the trend is now back to liberal use of natural carbohydrates in a balanced diet. There are, of course, many good reasons why you should eat generous amounts of fresh fruits, vegetables, and whole-grain products.

Carbohydrates Are Low in Calories

In addition to being rich in stomach-filling bulk in the form of water and fiber, natural carbohydrates are low in calories and rich in essential nutrients. Although carbohydrate foods do not contain all the essential amino acids (the building blocks of protein), the protein they supply in a balanced diet combines to form a complete protein that reduces your need for fat-rich animal protein.

On the new macro-nutrient diet, your calorie intake will be broken down into percentages of energy intake from carbohydrate, protein, and fat. *Carbohydrate*, however, is the principal fuel of the body. You need only enough fat to convey fat-soluble vitamins and to provide essential fatty acids. Protein is used primarily for the maintenance and repair of muscles and organs. In meeting the needs of your body, you need much more carbohydrate than protein, and fat should be kept to a minimum.

An excessive intake of any energy nutrient—carbohydrate, protein, or fat—can result in a buildup of body fat. Since fat has the highest concentration of calories, cutting down on dietary fat will greatly reduce calorie intake. But you still must be cautious about exceeding your calorie requirement in consuming other types of foods.

Prevent Disease with Carbohydrates

Keeping the animal fat in your diet to a minimum will help protect your heart and your blood vessels by reducing your intake of saturated fat and cholesterol. A diet high in natural carbohydrates will help prevent heart disease by *lowering* blood levels of triglycerides (fat) and cholesterol. Natural carbohydrates also improve glucose tolerance and reduce insulin requirements in diabetics.

Doctors have only recently discovered that a diet of fiber-rich natural carbohydrates is more beneficial for diabetics than the standard low-carbohydrate diet. According to *Dietary Goals for the United States*, "A high complex carbohydrate diet is important in the treatment of diabetics because it reduces the threat of atherosclerosis and hyperlipidema, which are common to diabetics, by lowering cholesterol and fat levels."

This is not to say, however, that it's all right to eat *refined* carbohydrates. Everyone, diabetic or not, should try to avoid consumption of refined sugars and processed carbohydrates. *Natural* carbohydrates have beneficial effects on blood sugar because of their water and fiber content. But when *refined* carbohydrates are eaten, they supply concentrated glucose that is absorbed so rapidly that there is a sudden and abnormal elevation in blood sugar. This triggers an overreaction from the pancreas, producing an excessive amount of insulin. As a result, blood sugar may fall or fluctuate abnormally, causing fatigue, mental confusion, and other symptoms of hypoglycemia (low blood sugar).

Pancreatic exhaustion resulting from overconsumption of refined carbohydrates may eventually lead to the development of diabetes. Persons already suffering from diabetes should avoid refined carbohydrates as if they were poison. It's important to remember that natural carbohydrates and refined carbohydrates are not the same. While you should *increase* your intake of natural carbohydrates, you should *avoid* refined carbohydrates.

Complex Carbohydrates Supply Essential Fiber

Natural carbohydrates are rich in a fiber called cellulose, which provides bulk that slows absorption of calories. Cellulose also holds water and sweeps the bowel clean. Refined carbohydrates, on the other hand, contain no fiber and are absorbed rapidly, leaving a sticky residue that clogs the bowel and feeds unfriendly colon bacteria. All carbohydrates supply glucose that your brain and your muscles use for fuel. But it would be much better to make sure that this fuel is supplied by *natural* carbohydrates that supply fiber and essential nutrients as well as glucose.

Contrary to popular opinion, natural carbohydrates, as a source of glucose, are *not* more fattening than protein and fat. Actually, a serving of a natural carbohydrate food contains *fewer* calories than an equal serving of an animal product. A baked potato, for example, contains fewer calories than a serving of beef. "Potatoes have had a very bad press," complained actress Loretta Swit. "They are a wonderful, nourishing vegetable—depending upon what you eat the rest of the day."

The new U.S. Dietary Goals advise us to reduce our intake of fat and increase our intake of natural carbohydrates, including potatoes. An increase in the consumption of complex carbohydrates, they contend, may provide a solution to America's nutritional problems. The authors of *Dietary Goals* explain that "One of the principal reasons for reducing the consumption of fat is to make a place in the diet for complex carbohydrates, which generally carry higher levels of micro-nutrients than fat without the complications of fat. . . . Furthermore, the high water content and bulk of fruits and vegetables and the bulk of whole grains can bring a longer lasting satisfaction of appetite more quickly than do foods high in fats and refined and processed sugars."

The Most Important Diet Discovery in Ten Years!

All foods supply calories. As you have learned, natural carbohydrates are more filling and less fattening and can be eaten in larger quantities than other types of foods. This has been demonstrated many times in actual dieting practices. The Chinese, for example, eat liberal amounts of rice, vegetables, and fruits in a high-carbohydrate diet. In fact, because of extensive consumption of rice, grains, sweet potatoes, and other natural carbohydrates, the average citizen of China gets about *80 percent* of daily energy needs from carbohydrate! Most of the remaining 20 percent of calories comes from protein. With the exception of a little vegetable oil used in stir frying, very little fat is consumed. Sweets are seldom eaten. As you might expect from what I have told you about natural carbohydrates, obesity is rare in China.

The vegetarian diet of Seventh Day Adventists is also high in carbohydrate. Blood studies indicate that serum levels of cholesterol and triglycerides among Adventists are lower than those of the average American.

You'll learn in Chapter 2 how to adjust your fat-burner throttle by dividing your calorie intake among the energy nutrients on a high-carbohydrate diet for permanent weight loss. The average person, however, can lose weight and maintain good health simply by observing the U.S. Dietary Goals. According to Consumer Guide (*Diets* '79), "The most important diet advanced in America in the last ten years has come from the U.S. Senate's Select Committee on Nutrition and Human Needs. *Dietary Goals for the United States* actually is not a diet, *per se*, but guidelines for a diet. Its principles consolidate the findings of the best nutritional research to date."

THE U.S. DIETARY GOALS

Here are the new U.S. Dietary Goals, revised and published in December of 1977.

1. To avoid overweight, consume only as much energy

(calories) as is expended; if overweight, decrease energy intake and increase energy expenditure.

2. Increase the consumption of complex carbohydrates and "naturally occurring" sugars from about 28 percent of energy intake to about 48 percent of energy intake.
3. Reduce the consumption of refined and processed sugars by about 45 percent to account for about 10 percent of total energy intake.
4. Reduce overall fat consumption from approximately 40 percent to about 30 percent of energy intake.
5. Reduce saturated fat consumption to account for about 10 percent of total energy intake; and balance that with polyunsaturated and monounsaturated fats, which should account for about 10 percent of energy intake each.
6. Reduce cholesterol consumption to about 300 milligrams a day.
7. Limit the intake of sodium by reducing the intake of salt to about 5 grams a day.

Translated into general rules for the average person to follow, the U.S. Dietary Goals suggest the following changes in food selection and preparation:

1. Increase consumption of fruits and vegetables and whole grains.
2. Decrease consumption of refined and other processed sugars and foods high in such sugars.
3. Decrease consumption of foods high in total fat, and partially replace saturated fats, whether obtained from animal or vegetable sources, with polyunsaturated fats.
4. Decrease consumption of animal fat, and choose meats, poultry, and fish which will reduce saturated fat intake.
5. Except for children, substitute low-fat and non-fat milk for whole milk, and low-fat dairy products for high-fat dairy products.
6. Decrease consumption of butterfat, eggs, and other high cholesterol sources. Some consideration should be given to easing the cholesterol goal for premenstrual women, young children, and the elderly in order to obtain the nutritional benefits of eggs in the diet.

7. Decrease consumption of salt and foods high in salt content.

These general rules apply to everyone, overweight or not. I would suggest, however, that you avoid refined and processed sugars and carbohydrates altogether if possible, substituting protein or natural carbohydrate. You'll learn more about how to do this in the next chapter. In the meantime, *you can begin reducing excess body fat simply by eliminating sugar, white flour, refined cereals, and other refined and processed foods from your diet and by selecting only natural foods from each of the seven basic food groups.*

Famous People Eat Simple Foods

John Beradino, a former professional baseball player turned actor, has kept his weight under control by eating only simple, basic foods. "I don't think I've picked up more than five or six pounds since I quit playing ball," he reported. "I eat the basic staples and cut out fat as much as possible. I don't live the Hollywood life, so I go home each night and eat my wife's home-cooked meals. She might have a roast with potatoes and string beans, for example. I like tuna, chicken, and fish. I snack on fruits."

Because of his good eating habits, John Beradino has never had to go on a strict diet.

Actor Ted Knight has found that all he has to do to keep his weight down is to avoid sugar and processed foods. "I don't have to go on a special diet to control my body weight," he explained. "I may have dropped 10 or 12 pounds over the past few years, but all I do is watch what I put into my system. I don't eat processed foods or desserts. I never use sugar."

TV actress Loretta Swit learned from experience how to feed her body. "I have learned over the years to listen to my body," Loretta explained. "The body has a way of telling us what we need. It's important to eat when you're hungry, for example. If you eat *natural* foods, you won't get into trouble. I don't eat junk foods. I don't think that you have a good, healthy body by accident. You are what you eat and you are what you do."

When I was collecting famous-person interviews for *Peter Lupus' Celebrity Body Book* (Parker), which I co-authored with actor Peter Lupus, I learned that most beautiful people eat fresh, natural foods in a simple diet. The material I gathered in preparing that book contributed greatly to the formulation of my macro-nutrient diet. You can eat like the beautiful people, and you, too, can be beautiful and healthy.

EAT AND ENJOY ON A MACRO-NUTRIENT DIET!

One of the first questions dieters ask about any new diet is "Will I get enough to eat?" I'm happy to report that on a macro-nutrient diet you'll be able to eat heartily while reducing excess body fat. One of the secrets of the success of a macro-nutrient diet is the high fiber and water content of the delicious natural carbohydrates you'll be allowed to eat. Many dieters are actually unable to eat all the food allowed on a macro-nutrient diet, even though they stay within certain calorie limitations. Natural macro-nutrient foods are wonderfully tasty, and their fiber content is so high that they are completely filling and totally satisfying. Furthermore, the great variety of flavors found in foods supplied by nature will make eating refreshing as well as delightfully pleasurable.

"I have never enjoyed eating so much," said Willard R., who lost 25 pounds in five weeks on a macro-nutrient diet. "After eating fresh, natural foods on a macro-nutrient diet, I could never go back to my old eating habits. Besides, I'm now so used to eating large amounts of natural carbohydrates that I won't want to substitute any other type of food. No other diet could ever replace my macro-nutrient diet!"

Nicholos C. echoed Willard's sentiments. "If I'm going to lose weight and keep it off," he leveled, "I'll have to be able to eat generous amounts and *enjoy* what I eat." Nicholos lost 76 pounds in six months—and that was two years ago. "I'm still eating well and enjoying what I eat," Nicholos reported, "and the fat has not come back."

This story has been told many times by persons who follow the macro-nutrient principles of dieting. You'll tell this story, too, after you have been on a macro-nutrient diet for a few months. And the basic foods you'll be eating will supply the nutrients you need for greater energy and more zestful living.

THE SEVEN BASIC FOOD GROUPS

The trend in recent years has been to reduce the seven basic food groups to four. In order to assure an adequate intake of natural carbohydrate with high levels of all the essential vitamins and minerals, I still prefer the *seven* food groups. In the four groups, fruits and vegetables are combined. Since both fruits and vegetables are carbohydrates, placing them in one group tends to reduce carbohydrate intake. Selecting from seven groups, however, will assure a greater intake of carbohydrate, since four of the groups are in the carbohydrate category. Try to eat something from each of these seven food groups each day:

1. Green and yellow vegetables (carbohydrate category)
2. Citrus fruit, tomatoes, and raw cabbage (carbohydrate category)
3. Potatoes and other vegetables and fruits (carbohydrate category)
4. Skimmed milk and skimmed milk products (protein category)
5. Lean meat, fish, eggs, skinned poultry, and dried peas and beans (protein category)
6. Whole-grain bread, cereal, and flour (carbohydrate category)
7. Butter, margarine, and vegetable oil (fat category)

Foods in the carbohydrate and protein category are never pure carbohydrate or pure protein. Vegetables and grains, for example, contain some protein. Meats are rich in saturated fat, while grains and vegetables supply important unsaturated fat. If you consume a variety of foods in a balanced diet, you won't have to worry about getting all of your protein from foods in the protein category or all of your fat from foods in the fat category. But you should use these categories in selecting foods in a balanced diet. It's important to eat a variety of foods to balance your intake of macro-nutrients.

Vitamins and minerals must also be supplied by a variety of foods. Generally, however, you should strive to get Vitamin A from green and yellow vegetables, Vitamin B from meats, Vitamin C from citrus fruits, Vitamin D from eggs and oils, Vitamin E from whole-grain products, and Vitamin F (essential fatty acids) from vegetable oil. You should be getting calcium from dairy products, iron from meats, and iodine from seafood. In a balanced diet, you'll also be getting some Vitamin C from fresh potatoes, some calcium from green leafy vegetables, and some Vitamin B_{12} from eggs and milk. So you won't be depending upon any single food to meet your requirements for a specific nutrient. No one food is indispensable in a properly balanced diet.

You'll learn more in Chapter 4 about how to get the vitamins and minerals you need from the foods you eat. In the meantime, you can assure an adequate intake of the essential nutrients by selecting fresh, natural foods from each of the basic food groups.

THE BASIC FOUR FOOD GROUPS

If you prefer to condense the seven food groups into four, use these food selections as a guide in planning your daily meals:

1. Two or more cups of skim milk or skim-milk products
2. Two or more servings of poultry, fish, or lean meat (with dry beans, dry peas, and nuts as alternatives)
3. Four or more servings of vegetables and fruits—including a citrus fruit, a dark-green or deep-yellow vegetable, and two servings of other fruits and vegetables, including potatoes
4. Four or more servings of whole-grain products (bread or cereal)

Fat should be kept to a minimum. Lean meats will supply all the fat you need, which will be balanced by the oils supplied by vegetables.

GENERAL RULES FOR HEALTHFUL EATING
ON A SLIMMING DIET

In order to simplify dieting procedures for persons who want to go on a slimming diet without measuring energy nutrients, I have formulated a few general rules that combine the U.S. Dietary

Goals with a few suggestions of my own. Try following these rules before going to a more restricted diet. Don't get in too big a hurry to lose weight. It may be better to condition your body by making a few general changes in your diet before cutting food portions too drastically. Besides, you might discover that you can lose weight simply by following a few basic rules.

If you are obese, or more than 20 pounds overweight, chances are you can begin to shed excess body fat by doing nothing more than cutting out refined foods and by eating less. Then, when you stop losing weight, or when your calorie intake exceeds the number of calories needed to reduce your existing weight, you can begin reducing your calorie intake by figuring calorie needs for your new weight goal. You'll learn how to do this in Chapter 3 when I tell you how to control your reducing power pedal.

In the meantime, *everyone, overweight or not, should observe the following general rules.*

1. Do not use sugar or eat foods containing sugar or white flour. Following this simple rule will eliminate candy, cake, pies, white bread, pastries, and other highly fattening foods. You can do without sweeteners other than fresh and dried fruits. Cereals, for example, can be sweetened with raisins and sliced fruit—or maybe a little honey in the case of hot cereal. (Since honey is sweeter than sugar, you'll use less honey than sugar.)

I do not recommend artificial sweeteners, since they may have harmful cumulative effects in the body. This means that you should not drink soft drinks, no matter how they are sweetened. At the present time, manufacturers of soft drinks use more sugar than any other industry. The average cola contains seven to 10 teaspoons of sugar! A 12-ounce can of cola, for example, contains about nine teaspoons of sugar.

If you do not limit your diet to fresh, natural foods, you can never be sure how much sugar or refined carbohydrate you are consuming. Canned foods often contain sugar. One tablespoon of catsup contains about one teaspoon of sugar. Most processed foods contain sugar or some other form of refined carbohydrate. One teaspoon of white sugar contains only about 15 calories. So an occasional teaspoon of sugar won't hurt you. But most people who use sugar don't stop with one or two teaspoons. If processed foods are eaten, large quantities of hidden sugar may be consumed. If

you don't make a special effort to eat natural foods and avoid consumption of sugar-sweetened foods, you may find it impossible to
control your weight. The average American, who is overweight
because of dietary indiscretion, consumes about 120 pounds of
sugar a year!

White flour, like white sugar, is a refined carbohydrate and
can be just as fattening as sugar. If you eat spaghetti, noodles,
pizza, and similar foods, select a variety made of whole-grain flour.
Spaghetti, for example, can be made with whole-wheat flour. Actress Barbara Feldon makes pizza crust from artichoke flour. Gloria
Swanson makes her own whole-wheat flour by grinding wheat kernels. Any health food store can supply you with a variety of whole-
grain flours for cooking and baking.

2. *Avoid processed foods whenever possible.* Some foods must
be processed to permit storage and shipping around the nation.
When you have a choice, however, you should always select a
fresh, natural food. Natural peanut butter, for example, contains
nothing but peanuts, but the hydrogenated variety may be loaded
with lard, saturated fat, sugar, preservatives, and other additives.
Many processed foods are so altered from their natural state that
they supply little more than calories. Processed cereals are converted from wholesome natural carbohydrate to refined carbohydrates that are deficient in fiber as well as nutrients. Try to avoid
such foods as powdered potatoes, white rice, fruit "drinks," and
manufactured snacks. You should also try to avoid cheeses and
meats that have been processed with added ingredients. Make it a
part of your life style to demand fresh, natural foods when you
snack as well as during meals.

Read the label on any packaged foods you purchase. Under
the new labeling law, ingredients are listed in descending order
according to weight. When you read the labels on processed cereals and snacks, you might be surprised to learn that *sugar* is often
the number one ingredient, followed by a long list of artificial
additives. Other sweeteners may be listed under such names as
sucrose, dextrose, fructose, and corn syrup. Fat may be listed as
butter, margarine, shortening, hydrogenated oil, vegetable oil, or
glycerides. Remember: the less sugar and fat you consume the
better.

3. Eat fish, eggs, skinned poultry, fresh fruits and vegetables, raw salads, whole-grain breads and cereals, and cottage cheese and yogurt made from skim milk. These foods will provide low-fat sources of all the essential nutrients. Always cut away visible fat on meats—and remove the skin from poultry. Remember, however, that some "lean" meats may be as much as 40 percent fat. So don't eat too much meat, especially red meats. Pork is higher in fat (and calories) than most meats. Veal is generally low in fat. Fish and poultry contain the least fat of all and are just as rich in protein as red meats, though less rich in iron. (Oysters contain more iron than meat, poultry, *or* fish!)

Whole-grain products and green leafy vegetables will help complete your iron requirement, as will fruits, especially dried fruits. But if you don't eat much red meat, try to eat liver at least once a week.

4. Do not use fats or oils in cooking. Remember that in addition to providing a highly concentrated source of calories, an excessive amount of fat in the diet may contribute to the development of cancer, atherosclerosis, and other diseases. When you overheat fat or oil in cooking, the fatty acids break down to become even more carcinogenic—and they may irritate the intestinal tract.

Cooking with fat or oil greatly increases the calorie content of a food. Potato chips, for example, are 40 percent fat compared to 0.1 percent fat in a baked potato. You don't have to cook with fat. You can broil meats and steam vegetables. Fruits and some vegetables should be eaten raw. You'll learn more in Chapter 4 about how to cook the low-fat way to reduce calorie intake as well as to preserve nutrients.

5. Increase the amount of fiber in your diet by eating more whole-grain products and raw fruits and vegetables and by adding unprocessed miller's bran to breakfast cereal and homemade bread. You can probably get all the fiber you need from whole-grain products and vegetables if your diet is properly balanced. Remember, however, that overcooking a vegetable diminishes its fiber content by destroying its cellulose. So cook your vegetables as little as possible, and eat something *raw* each day.

You can add additional fiber to your diet by adding miller's bran to foods. Unfortunately, the phytates in bran tend to interfere with the absorption of calcium, iron, and other minerals. It might be best, therefore, to add bran only to cereals and homemade bread. Chapter 6 will tell you how to use bran and other food fibers for more rapid weight loss.

6. *Use skim milk, vegetable juices, and water as beverages.* Drink *water* when you are thirsty. Unsalted bouillon and Perrier water flavored with lemon juice also make good low-calorie beverages. Remember that vegetable juices are lower in calories than fruit juices. With the exception of your morning glass of fruit juice with breakfast, you should always eat the whole fruit rather than squeeze it for juice. The pulp of fruit provides filling bulk that will reduce your appetite for more fattening foods.

Robert Pine of "CHiPs" and his wife, actress Gwynne Gilford, make a healthful "soft drink" by mixing equal amounts of grape juice and Perrier water. Since Perrier water naturally contains carbon dioxide, it fizzes like a carbonated drink. When you are at a cocktail party and you want to avoid high-calorie alcoholic drinks, you can bluff your way with Perrier water or fruit juice. Or you can follow Dr. Joyce Brothers' example and mix club soda with lemon juice. I personally prefer tomato juice with a twist of lemon. If you enjoy nightclubbing without alcohol, don't be reluctant to order tomato juice or fruit juice if that's what you want.

7. *Use one tablespoon of cold-pressed vegetable oil on a green salad each day.* This will supply the unsaturated fat you need to balance the saturated fat in your diet. And on a low-fat diet you may need the oil to aid absorption of fat-soluble vitamins. Remember, however, that heating a vegetable oil destroys its essential fatty acids. So don't depend upon heated or cooked oils for nutritional balance.

Safflower oil is richest in linoleic acid, the fatty acid most essential for humans. But any vegetable oil is fine. You can mix vegetable oil with vinegar or lemon juice for use as a salad dressing.

8. *Eat slowly at mealtime.* Stop eating when you are comfortably full. If you'll get up from the table a little hungry, chances are you won't be hungry half an hour or so later. It takes about 20 minutes for circulating blood sugar and other nutrients to reach the appetite centers in your brain. So don't ever try to completely satisfy your hunger while eating. If you do, and you eat rapidly, you'll overeat.

Behavior modification, or attention to when, where, and how you eat, can be just as important as what you eat and how you prepare your foods when you are on a slimming diet. You'll find many tips on behavior modification in Chapter 10.

9. *Satisfy your craving for sweets by eating fresh and dried fruits for desserts following meals.* You should never eat sweets of any kind between meals or before meals, lest you kill your appetite for more nutritious foods. When you do eat sweets, they should be in the form of fruits, dates, and other natural foods. Such sweets will provide fiber as well as nutrients. Artificial sweets contain only empty calories that will artificially stimulate your appetite, resulting in overindulgence.

10. *If you feel hungry between meals, snack on raw vegetables, baked chicken, or a little plain yogurt or uncreamed cottage cheese with fresh fruit.* Don't ever succumb to the temptation to eat sweets, pastries, and other processed foods between meals. This may only lead to a blood sugar problem that might escalate into fat-building eating binges. If you do eat between meals, eat something that is low in sugar and fat, such as fruit and yogurt. Then eat less at mealtime. Studies indicate that people who eat small but frequent meals tend to store less fat than persons who eat large, irregular meals.

If you suffer from between-meal weakness, fatigue, and shakiness that you suspect might be the result of low blood sugar, be sure to study the material on hypoglycemia in Chapter 7.

A SAMPLE NATURAL-FOOD DIET PLAN

The remaining chapters of this book will discuss the special approach of my macro-nutrient diet. In the meantime, here is a sample diet plan for low-fat, low-calorie meals made up entirely of natural foods. You can eat generous amounts of all vegetables that are prepared without grease or oil.

Breakfast

One egg *or* a serving of lean ham, Canadian bacon, or veal.
One slice of whole-grain bread with a cup of skim milk *or* a whole-grain cereal with skim milk. (Cereal may be sweetened with dried or fresh fruit.)
One piece of citrus fruit *or* a glass of fruit juice.

Lunch

Fish *or* skinned chicken *or* a lean meat of your choice. (Remember that chicken and fish are lowest in saturated fat.)
One dark green vegetable *or* one deep yellow vegetable.
One other vegetable of your choice.
One slice of whole-grain bread *or* a serving of coarse corn bread.
One cup of vegetable juice, water, or skim milk as a beverage with meal.
For dessert: Melon, fresh fruit, or dried fruit. (Unprocessed cheese with a serving of fresh fruit makes a satisfying dessert.)

Dinner

A serving of the same meat dish you had at lunch *or* a serving of cottage cheese, pot cheese, or farmer's cheese.
A fresh, raw vegetable salad laced with a tablespoon of cold-pressed vegetable oil and lemon juice.
A slice of whole-grain bread or a few whole-grain wafers.
A cup of vegetable juice or a cup of skim milk. (Make sure that you have two cups of skim milk or its equivalent each day.)

If you have a blender, you can liquify whole fruits and vegetables to make beverages that are filling, low in calories, and high in fiber. Chilled, blended vegetables make great between-meal snacks. Of course, plain water has no calories at all. Drink plenty of water.

TAKING THE IGNORANCE OUT OF DIETING

Many persons fail in their dieting efforts because they do not understand what they are doing. They are simply unable to adjust their diet to meet their particular needs. Milton D., for example, was not often able to eat at home. And since he did not know how to balance his intake of carbohydrate, protein, and fat, he could not control his calorie intake, especially when eating out. "Since I've been on your macro-nutrient diet," Milton observed, "I have been able to select and balance my foods while traveling as well as at home. I have learned how to distinguish one type of food from another. I finally know *how* to diet! I lost 20 pounds in three months with no trouble at all. And I haven't gained an ounce of it back."

Dolly T. did not know how to diet, either. Instead of learning how to eat properly, she turned to fads. "The simplest way to lose weight," she argued, "is to quit eating." So Dolly went to a hypnotist who gave her a mimeographed low-carbohydrate diet and "hypnotized" her to diminish her desire for food. When I saw Dolly in my office, she was depressed, fatigued, and suffering from chronic headache. Her blood sugar was below normal and her system was poisoned with ketones.

Taking Dolly off her bad diet resulted in a quick weight gain as her body quickly restored lost water. But after she became accustomed to eating properly, she once again began to lose weight. "I'm losing only about two pounds a week," Dolly reported. "But I feel great and I'm eating all kinds of good foods. I'd much rather lose weight slowly and permanently than lose faster on a bad diet that makes me feel bad."

Once you've experienced the physical well-being of losing weight on a good diet, you won't be tempted by bad diets. You cannot replace sensible eating with hypnotism, ear staples, mono diets, and other fads. Protect your health and prevent embarrassment by learning how to eat properly so that you won't be exploited by dangerous fads.

Weight Loss May Vary

Just because Dolly lost only two pounds a week doesn't mean that you can't lose more weight faster. You can control your reducing power pedal (calorie intake) and adjust your fat-burner throttle (energy nutrient sources) to govern rate of weight loss to suit yourself. Ernie D., for example, lost an average of four pounds a week on a macro-nutrient diet. "I lost 16 pounds in a month by cutting my calorie intake and concentrating on natural carbohydrates," he explained. "I've never been on a reducing diet that allowed me to eat so much food!"

Marsha U. lost an average of five pounds a week during one month on a 1,200 calorie macro-nutrient diet. "I lost a total of 20 pounds," Marsha reported with a wide smile. "I never before lost that much weight on a diet. It must have something to do with the *type* of foods I've been eating."

Yes, it did have something to do with the type of food Marsha was eating. When you switch to a diet of fresh, natural foods, chances are you'll begin to shed excess body fat immediately, even if you eat plentifully. A *low-calorie* diet of fresh, natural foods holds many surprises in a reducing program. So even when your calorie calculations indicate that you can expect to lose only two or three pounds a week, you might actually lose four or five pounds a week if you eat natural foods, increase your intake of food fiber, and stay physically active.

You'll learn more about the variables in dieting in other chapters of this book. The next two chapters will tell you how to force more rapid weight loss by controlling your reducing power pedal and by adjusting your fat-burner throttle. So keep reading!

SUMMARY

1. *Fad diets that result in a rapid but temporary weight loss often dehydrate the body because of inadequate carbohydrate intake.*

2. *You can shed excess body fat* permanently *by including generous amounts of* natural *carbohydrates in a balanced diet.*

3. *According to the new U.S. Dietary Goals, the problem of overweight in America can be solved by reducing our intake of fat and processed foods and by* increasing *our intake of complex (natural) carbohydrates.*

4. *Natural carbohydrates are low in calories and high in water, fiber, and nutrients.*

5. *Every healthy American should consume at least 100 grams of natural carbohydrate and 60 grams of low-fat protein each day.*

6. *According to the new U.S. Dietary Goals, 58 percent of energy intake should come from carbohydrate, 30 percent from fat, and 12 percent from protein.*

7. *Most people could lose weight simply by refusing to eat sugar, white flour, and other refined carbohydrates.*

8. *Selecting foods from the basic seven or basic four food groups in recommended servings will automatically balance your diet if you select only fresh, natural foods.*

9. *Beverages with meals should be limited to unsweetened juices, skim milk, and water.*

10. *Such general measures as eating low-fat natural foods prepared without grease or oil may be effective in reducing excess body fat.*

2

How to Adjust Your Fat-Burner Throttle on an Effortless Slimming Program with Macro-Nutrient Foods

If you fail to lose weight after a couple of weeks following the general measures outlined in Chapter 1, you'll have to control your calorie intake and measure food portions of carbohydrate, protein, and fat. I have already told you that the new U.S. Dietary Goals recommend that 48 percent of your total calorie intake should come from complex (natural) carbohydrate, 10 percent from sugar and refined carbohydrate, 30 percent from fat, and 12 percent from protein. On the new macro-nutrient *slimming diet,* in which calorie intake will be reduced for weight loss, you'll be adjusting your fat-burner throttle by substituting *protein* for the 10 percent refined and processed sugars. Bringing your protein intake up to about 22 percent of your total energy intake will assure adequate protein on a low-calorie diet.

On a higher-calorie *maintenance diet,* which you use to maintain your ideal body weight, you should substitute *natural carbohydrate* for the 10 percent refined and processed sugars, bringing your intake of natural carbohydrate up to about 58 percent of your energy intake. In order to control your fat-burner throttle effectively, you should make sure that fat never supplies more than 30 percent of your energy intake. In fact, the less fat you consume the better.

HOW TO ADJUST ENERGY NUTRIENTS ON
A 1,200 CALORIE DIET

In order to determine what percentages of your calories are coming from carbohydrate, protein, and fat, you'll first have to measure your calorie intake. If you go on a 1,200 calorie diet, you can then break-up the 1,200 calories into the recommended percentages. For example, on a low-calorie *slimming diet*, 48 percent of 1,200 calories from carbohydrate equals *576 carbohydrate calories;* 22 percent of 1,200 calories from protein equals *264 protein calories;* and 30 percent of 1,200 calories from fat equals *360 fat calories.*

We know that carbohydrate supplies four calories per gram, protein four calories per gram, and fat nine calories per gram. This means that 576 carbohydrate calories divided by four equal *144 grams of carbohydrate;* 264 protein calories divided by four equal *66 grams of protein;* and 360 fat calories divided by nine equal *40 grams of fat.*

Thus, *on a 1,200 calorie diet, you should be taking in about 144 grams of carbohydrate, 66 grams of protein, and 40 grams of fat.*

To select the correct amount of food in grams, you'll first have to decide what foods you want to eat from each of the basic four or basic seven food groups and then measure these foods in grams. The Table of Nutritive Values in Chapter 12 will give you the gram weight of proper food portions and tell you how much of the food is carbohydrate, protein, and fat. For example, one cup of nonfat (skim) milk supplies about 90 calories with 12 grams of carbohydrate, nine grams of protein, and a trace of fat. If you add up the calories and the grams of carbohydrate, protein, and fat supplied by the foods in each meal, you can quickly calculate the percentage of calories being supplied by each type of energy nutrient. (Remember that carbohydrate supplies four calories per gram, protein four calories per gram, and fat nine calories per gram.)

HOW TO ADJUST ENERGY NUTRIENTS ON
A 2,000 CALORIE DIET

On a 1,200 calorie slimming diet, I recommend that you get about 48 percent of your calories from natural carbohydrate and about 22 percent from protein in order to assure an adequate intake of protein—at least 60 grams.

The recommended daily allowance of protein for the average adult is about 55 grams daily, depending upon height, weight, and sex. The average male between the ages of 23 and 50, for example, who weighs 154 pounds needs about 56 grams of protein daily compared to 46 grams for a female of the same age who weighs about 128 pounds. And to maintain their weight, the male must take in 2,700 calories daily and the female about 2,000 calories daily. When your diet is high in natural carbohydrate, you can take in considerably more than 100 grams of carbohydrate and still reduce excess body fat if your calorie output exceeds your calorie intake.

On a diet of 2,000 calories or more, which will be a maintenance diet for some and a reducing diet for others, 58 percent of calories from natural carbohydrate and 12 percent of calories from protein will provide adequate protein.

The Mathematics of a 2,000 Calorie Diet

Since a balanced higher-calorie diet will supply more protein than a balanced lower-calorie diet, you can get adequate protein from 2,000 calories or more simply by following the percentages recommended by the new U.S. Dietary Goals. But remember that I recommend that you *substitute natural carbohydrate for the 10 percent sugar and processed carbohydrates so that carbohydrates supply about 58 percent of your total intake of calories.*

Here's how the math looks when figuring energy nutrient percentages on a 2,000 calorie diet:

Step 1: *Recommended energy intake percentages*
    58% natural carbohydrate
    12% protein
    30% fat

Step 2: *Calories to be supplied by energy nutrients*
    58% of 2,000 calories = 1,160 carbohydrate calories
    12% of 2,000 calories = 240 protein calories
    30% of 2,000 calories = 600 fat calories

Step 3: *Calories per gram of energy nutrients*
Carbohydrate: 4 calories per gram
Protein: 4 calories per gram
Fat: 9 calories per gram

Step 4: *Calories translated into grams of energy nutrients*
1,160 carbohydrate calories divided by 4 = 290 grams of carbohydrates
240 protein calories divided by 4 = 60 grams of protein
600 fat calories divided by 9 = 66 grams of fat

Step 5: *Grams of energy nutrients translated into food servings*
Now all you have to do is select enough food from each of the basic four or seven food groups to supply the recommended grams of energy nutrients. You can do this by consulting the Table of Nutritive Values in Chapter 12.

Once you understand how to break your calorie requirement into the recommended percentages of energy nutrients, and then how to translate calories into grams of energy nutrients (or grams of energy nutrients into calories) by using the Table in Chapter 12, you can develop your own diet with the foods you like best and you can select the number of calories best suited to your particular body weight. You won't have to follow someone else's diet that tells you exactly what to eat at every meal seven days a week.

You'll learn in Chapter 3 how to determine the number of calories you should take in each day in order to control your reducing power pedal so that you can attain or maintain a body weight that is best for you. "If you maintain your ideal weight within half a pound," advises actor Lyle Waggoner, "you can usually maintain your health."

PATIENT, LONG-RANGE DIETING IS BEST

Sue E. was 105 pounds overweight. "I could never lose that much weight," she complained with an air of resignation. "I've been fat as long as I can remember." I explained to Sue that she could shed her excess fat by losing only a few pounds at a time. "Don't think about dropping 105 pounds of fat," I advised. "Think only about weekly weight goals. Any goal can be overwhelming if you think of the whole thing at once."

Sue took my advice and concentrated only on losing a pound or two at a time rather than the entire 105 pounds. And she thought in terms of months rather than days. She lost 80 pounds in 10 months! "My weight loss has been so gradual and so easy that my weight goal of 135 pounds is going to be a snap," she said confidently.

If you'll be patient and set a series of long-range goals in your reducing program, you, too, can reach your ultimate goal one step and one pound at a time—with no strain at all.

How Gloria Ate Heartily and Lost 17 Pounds on a Macro-Nutrient Diet

Gloria B., at five feet five inches in height and 34 years of age, was an average American woman, except that she weighed 145 pounds rather than the recommended 128 pounds. Gloria needed to lose 17 pounds, but she didn't want to starve herself. Since about 2,000 calories a day would be needed to maintain her recommended weight of 128 pounds, she would have to take in *less* than 2,000 calories a day in order to force her body to burn stored fat. "If I could lose one pound a week," she said, "I could slim down in time for my summer vacation."

To lose one pound a week, Gloria would have to take in 500 fewer calories a day then she would need to maintain her recommended weight (see Chapter 3). This means that she could lose adequate weight on a generous diet that supplies about 1,500 calories a day.

Using the sample 1,200+ calorie diet outlined in this chapter, with two daily between-meal snacks of fresh fruit with eight ounces of uncreamed cottage cheese or plain yogurt, Gloria lost 17 pounds in four months without going hungry. "I had more than enough to eat," she reported with amazement. "I lost a little over a pound a week as promised, and I really couldn't tell that I was on a diet—quite the contrary."

If Gloria had limited her food intake to 1,200 calories daily instead of 1,500, she would have lost nearly two pounds a week. But she preferred to eat more and lose slowly in reaching her weight goal.

A big, large-framed, moderately active man who should normally weigh about 190 pounds but who weighs 240 pounds could easily lose a pound a week on a daily intake of 2,350 calories, since 2,850 calories would be needed to maintain his recommended weight (see Chapter 3). It would take him about a year to lose 50 pounds. Reducing his daily calorie intake to 1,850 calories would result in a loss of *two* pounds a week, with a total loss of about 50 pounds in six months. An intake of only 1,200 calories would result in a loss of more than three pounds a week. Weight loss in every instance would, of course, be *greater* if diet were combined with an exercise program.

Obviously, if you know how to figure your calorie requirement, *as explained in the next chapter,* you can control your calorie intake, thus controlling your reducing power pedal, so that you lose weight gradually and permanently with good eating habits. In the meantime, you should learn how to develop a diet with the recommended percentages of energy nutrients.

Practically anyone can lose weight on a 1,200 calorie diet. Most of the diets prescribed by doctors and dieticians for reducing purposes supply *at least* 1,200 calories. If you want a good, basic reducing diet, try my 1,200+ calorie diet.

HOW TO DEVELOP A 1,200+ CALORIE DIET

In providing you with a sample 1,200 calorie diet, I have listed the types of foods (from the basic food groups) that I generally recommend. If you prefer, you may select favorite foods from the basic food groups listed in Chapter 1. Just make sure that you at least meet the requirements outlined in the basic four food groups. For example, it doesn't matter which vegetables you eat as long as you have two servings of yellow and green vegetables and two servings of other vegetables. You should have one serving of your favorite citrus fruit and two servings of other fruits. It's important to make sure that your diet is balanced with the recommended variety of foods.

The following foods divided into three meals a day will supply a little more than 1,200 calories. It doesn't matter how you arrange food selections as long as you divide them into three or more meals. (Table 2-1.) I'll provide you with a sample three-meal menu later in this chapter.

Using the totals in Table 2-1 (1,275 calories, 68 grams of protein, 40 grams of fat, and 177 grams of carbohydrate), you can quickly calculate the percentage of calories coming from each of the energy nutrients.

68 grams of protein × 4 calories per gram = 272 calories

40 grams of fat × 9 calories per gram = 360 calories

177 grams of carbohydrate × 4 calories per gram = 708 calories

You'll notice that adding the number of calories obtained by multiplying calories per gram equals 1,340 calories, 65 more than you get by adding the calorie values given on food charts. Obviously, it's not possible to figure the *exact* number of calories supplied by food servings. *Any figures you use are approximate*, and that's all you need to figure energy-nutrient percentages.

GRAMS

	Calories	Protein	Fat	Carbohydrate
2 cups skim milk	180	18	trace	24
1 large egg	80	6	6	trace
3 ounces broiled fish or chicken	115	20	3	0
1 stalk cooked broccoli	45	6	1	8
1 cup cooked carrots	45	1	trace	10
1 medium baked potato	90	3	trace	21
1 cup cooked cabbage	30	2	trace	6
1 orange	65	1	trace	16
1 apple	70	trace	trace	18
1 peach	35	1	trace	10
2 slices whole wheat bread	120	6	2	24
2 shredded wheat biscuits	180	4	2	40
1 tablespoon butter	100	trace	12	trace
1 tablespoon vegetable oil	120	0	14	0
	1,275	68	40	177

Table 2-1

HOW TO CALCULATE ENERGY-NUTRIENT PERCENTAGES

To determine the percentage of calories obtained from each type of energy nutrient, divide the diet's total number of calories into each of the protein, fat, and carbohydrate totals. For example, the total number of calories, 1,340, divided into the 272 calories supplied by protein reveals that you are getting 20 percent of your calories from protein. With 360 calories coming from fat and 708 calories coming from carbohydrate, you are getting 27 percent of your calories from fat and 53 percent from carbohydrate. All these figures fall within the range recommended by the new U.S. Dietary Goals.

If your percentage figures show that you are getting too much fat or too little protein or carbohydrate, you can adjust your food selections accordingly. Of course, it's not necessary to take in energy nutrients in the exact amounts recommended in *Dietary Goals*. Just try to approximate them as closely as you can.

When you want to increase the number of calories in your diet, you should add some natural carbohydrate, such as vegetables, and some low-fat protein, such as fish or cottage cheese. If you need some additional fat, you can eat lean meat rather than fish or poultry. But remember that it's usually best to keep your intake of fat as low as possible. And remember that the unsaturated fat supplied by fish and poultry is more healthful than the saturated fat supplied by meat. Since meats normally contain fat, you'll get all the saturated fat you need from "lean" meats.

You can look over the Table of Nutritive Values in Chapter 12 and pick the foods that supply the calories and the energy nutrients you need most. Make sure that you eat something from all the basic food groups, however, as recommended in Chapter 1. Try to balance your intake of animal fat and vegetable fat. After you have determined your calorie requirement with the formula revealed in Chapter 3, you may simply decrease or increase servings of the basic foods according to their calorie content.

Remember that it's always a good idea to take a multiple vitamin-and-mineral supplement when your diet supplies less than 2,000 calories.

SAMPLE THREE-MEAL MENU

Here's a sample three-meal 1,200 calorie menu that actually supplies about 1,270 calories with 147 grams of carbohydrate, 94 grams of protein, and 34 grams of fat. About 46 percent of the calories are coming from carbohydrate, 30 percent from protein, and 24 percent from fat. (See Table 2-2.)

Selection of these foods according to their calorie content as listed on a food chart adds up to 1,185 calories. But when you add up the grams of carbohydrate, protein, and fat supplied by these foods and multiply calories per gram, you end up with 1,270 calories. Since calorie values are approximate, they will always vary slightly from listed values when figured in calories per gram.

	Calories	Protein	Fat	Carbohydrate
GRAMS				
Breakfast				
1 cup orange juice	110	2	1	26
1 egg	80	6	6	trace
1 slice whole wheat bread	60	3	1	12
1 pat of butter	35	trace	4	trace
1 cup coffee				
Lunch				
1 cup uncreamed cottage cheese	170	34	1	5
2 large lettuce leaves	10	1	trace	2
1 tomato	40	2	1	9
1 slice whole wheat bread	60	3	1	12
1 cup skim milk	90	9	trace	12
1 apple	70	trace	trace	18
Dinner				
2.5 ounces lean beef	140	22	5	0
1 cup cooked, diced beets	55	2	trace	12
2 lettuce leaves	10	1	trace	12
6 slices cucumber	5	trace	trace	2
1 tablespoon vegetable oil	120	trace	14	trace
1 tablespoon vinegar	trace	trace	0	1
1 cup skim milk	90	9	trace	12
2 dried apricot halves	40	trace	trace	12

Table 2-2

Remember that you may use the Chart of Nutritive Values in Chapter 12 to select the foods you like best in developing your own low-calorie balanced diet. The number of calories you choose to take in will depend upon your weight goal. So be sure to read Chapter 3 for instructions in controlling your reducing power pedal.

You'll find more sample menus in Chapter 11.

Special Note on Meat

Since red meats are rich in saturated fat and cholesterol, you should not eat them too often. It's better to eat fish or poultry. If you prefer not to eat the flesh of creatures, you should be sure to include low-fat milk and milk products (such as cottage cheese) and eggs in your diet. Limiting your diet to fruits, vegetables, and whole-grain products on a strictly carbohydrate or vegetarian diet would lead to deficiencies in calcium, iron, zinc, riboflavin, and Vitamin B_{12}. Combining grains and legumes in a vegetarian diet can supply a complete protein, but protein from animal products will supply adequate protein as well as Vitamin B_{12} and other essential nutrients. You'll learn more about how to get the nutrients you need from the foods you eat when you read Chapter 4. In the meantime, make sure that you eat something from each of the basic four groups each day. If you tend to be a vegetarian, Chapter 5 will be of special interest to you.

YOU ARE UNIQUE

It's important to understand that not everyone can follow the same 1,200 calorie diet or the same 2,000 calorie diet. The amount of food you need to supply the calories and the nutrients you need for the best of health while reducing excess body fat depends upon your activity level and your approximate ideal weight as determined by your height and the size of your frame. This is why I have given you only a couple of sample diets consisting of basic foods. You should select the foods you like best and then adjust your calorie intake according to your desired weight.

All you have to do to raise a 1,200 calorie diet to a 1,500 or 1,800 calorie diet is to add servings of whole-grain bread, your favorite vegetable, a little extra fish or poultry, and maybe a little more fruit. According to the Table of Nutritive Value of Foods in Chapter 12, for example, one slice of whole-grain bread (60 calories), one ear of corn (140 calories), three ounces of broiled chicken (115 calories), and one banana (100 calories) will supply an additional 415 low-fat calories.

When increasing the calorie content of your diet, be sure to keep your diet balanced by selecting a variety of foods. You may simply eat a little more of all the types of foods listed in the 1,200 calorie diet.

How Sandra Lost Weight by Eating More

Sandra T. was on a 1,200 calorie diet prescribed by her family physician. She was losing less than one pound a week. The reason, it seems, was that her diet was made up largely of processed and overcooked foods. When she limited her food selections to fresh, natural foods, often uncooked, she lost two to three pounds a week. Even with the inclusion of larger amounts of raw fruits and vegetables, Sandra continued to lose two or three pounds a week. "I've figured up my calorie intake," she said a few weeks after changing her diet, "and I've found that I'm taking in *more* than 1,200 calories a day. Yet, I'm losing twice as much weight as I did on my original 1,200 calorie diet."

One reason for Sandra's new success in dieting was the fact that she was eating more natural carbohydrates. The low-calorie bulk supplied by fresh fruits and vegetables provided twice as much food with only a few more calories. Furthermore, the calories supplied by these foods were more than offset by an increased intake of dietary fiber.

"I lost 10 pounds in one month," Sandra noted with disbelief. "And I just love all the fruits and vegetables I'm eating!"

You, too, will discover that a diet rich in natural carbohydrate is less fattening than a diet that allows consumption of refined carbohydrates. And because natural carbohydrates are so rich in water and fiber, you'll be able to eat more and still reduce excess body fat. Chapter 6 will reveal the secret of natural carbohydrate's effectiveness as a diet food.

KEEP YOUR STOMACH FULL WITH
MACRO-NUTRIENT FOODS

If you eat fresh, natural foods with emphasis on complex car-bohydrates, you'll discover that it takes a large amount of food to add up to 2,000 calories. In fact, many people have difficulty eating the quantity of food required to supply 2,000 or more calories on a maintenance diet. This is one reason why so many people lose weight on a low-fat natural foods diet even if they do not count calories. And when 58 percent of energy intake comes from natural carbohydrates, the bulk supplied by such foods is filling as well as low in calories. A baked potato, for example, supplies only about 90 calories while a 2½ ounce serving of *lean* beef supplies 140 calories. Without the fat trimmed away, a three-ounce serving of beef supplies 245 calories!

Most of the fat in meat is hidden, which means that many meats that appear to be lean may contain as much as 40 percent fat. This is one reason why it's difficult to measure your fat intake when you eat large amounts of meat.

Even fruits, which have a reputation for being high in sugar, are low in calories compared to meat and other non-carbohydrate foods. An apple, for example, contains only 70 calories and an orange about 65 calories. Because of the amount of fiber and water in these fruits, they supply twice as much bulk as a serving of beef that weighs only half as much as the fruit yet supplies more than three times as many calories. An orange weighs about 180 grams with 65 calories while a three-ounce serving of beef weighs only 85 grams with 245 calories.

Thus, *servings of fruits and vegetables and other natural car-bohydrates are generally twice as filling and one third as fattening as servings of animal products that contain fat.* So the next time someone tells you that fresh fruit is fattening, you can counter by saying that the odds are three to one in favor of the fruit.

Actor Gavin MacLeod, star of the TV series "Love Boat," lost 80 pounds of fat by increasing his intake of fruits and vegetables in a high-carbohydrate diet that included eggs and fish for protein.

How to Keep Your Diet Balanced for a Lifetime

You'll learn in the next chapter that it takes about 15 calories per pound of body weight to maintain your ideal weight if you are

moderately active. Once your body weight is down where you want
it to be, you can discontinue the low-calorie diet and take in more
calories by eating a little more of something from all the basic food
groups. You'll have to raise your calorie intake up to the level
needed to *maintain* your weight. The emphasis will continue to be
placed on natural carbohydrate. The type of foods you eat won't
change, just the amount. No reducing diet will be permanently
effective if you cannot continue to eat the same kind of foods you
ate to reduce your weight. Persons who eliminate basic foods or eat
only one type of food to reduce body weight usually regain the lost
weight when the diet is discontinued.

If you want to get rid of excess body fat permanently, you'll
have to learn how to eat *properly*. You can lose weight just as
effectively on a *balanced* low-calorie diet as on a fad diet that
eliminates essential foods. So if you're going to go to the trouble of
dieting, you might as well do it right and adopt a method that you
can follow for a lifetime. This means educating yourself in the
fundamentals of nutrition and then using a little common sense in
applying nutritional guides—as you'll do on the new macro-
nutrient diet.

MAKE YOUR DIET MORE EFFECTIVE BY EXERCISING

If you want to make your slimming diet more effective, you
should exercise as much as possible. The calories you burn in
physical activity, combined with the calorie deficit in your diet,
will add up to more weight loss than you could possibly attain by
diet alone, especially if you follow a good, safe diet. Any kind of
physical activity, such as washing the car or raking the yard, burns
calories. Try to participate in some form of recreational exercise
each day. Tennis, swimming, riding a bicycle, jumping a rope, and
similar activities, for example, are especially useful in reducing
excess body fat.

Persons who love to eat often exercise so that they can lose
weight by exercising rather than by dieting. But it's still important
to eat fresh, natural foods in a balanced diet. *Combining* exercise
with a good diet will improve your physical appearance as well as
speed weight loss, even while eating more. See *Peter Lupus'
Celebrity Body Book* (Parker Publishing Company) for guidance in
the use of exercise for weight loss and body shaping.

Malcolm B. lost 20 pounds during the first month on a macro-nutrient diet combined with exercise. "I play a little tennis three or four times a week," Malcolm said, "and I swim a couple of times a week. But I didn't really start losing my body fat until I changed my eating habits. My macro-nutrient diet has made the difference. I'm a new man! I'm 40 pounds lighter than I was five months ago, and my friends tell me that I look great. I plan to continue eating this way as long as I live."

One look at Malcolm was enough to convince anyone that he was eating right. You, too, will be your own best example when you eat properly and exercise regularly. At 51 years of age and 180 pounds, I have no trouble controlling my body weight with my macro-nutrient diet. You won't, either, if you follow the guidelines of this book.

SUMMARY

1. On a macro-nutrient reducing *diet, about 48 percent of your calorie intake will come from natural carbohydrate, 22 percent from protein, and 30 percent from fat.*

2. On a higher-calorie maintenance *diet, about 58 percent of your calorie intake should come from natural carbohydrate, with 12 percent from protein and 30 percent from fat.*

3. *Since one gram of carbohydrate supplies four calories, one gram of protein four calories, and one gram of fat nine calories, you can measure your intake of energy nutrients by consulting a table giving the gram and calorie values of foods.*

4. *If dieting gets too complicated, just try to get one third of your calories from each of the three energy components of food: carbohydrate, protein, and fat.*

5. *A reducing diet should never go below 1,200 calories.*

6. *Diets that supply less than 2,000 calories should be supplemented with vitamins and minerals.*

7. *You can eat the foods you like best as long as you select something from each basic food group each day.*

8. *Once you determine the approximate number of calories you need to take in, you can divide the calories into the recommended percentage of energy nutrients.*

9. *Remember that you can lose excess body fat faster by combining diet and exercise.*

10. *In order to control your calorie intake to maintain a desirable body weight, you'll have to know how to determine your calorie requirement—so be sure to read the next chapter.*

3

How to Control Your
Reducing Power Pedal to Attain
an Attractive, Ideal Body Weight
with Macro-Nutrient Foods

Long before the U.S. Dietary Goals were published, I had learned from experience that restricting fats and refined carbohydrates and including generous amounts of whole grains and fresh fruits and vegetables in a balanced diet is the most healthful and the least fattening way to eat. I also found that most people can reduce excess body fat by following a few general rules such as those outlined in Chapter 1. Simply increasing your intake of natural carbohydrates while reducing your intake of other types of foods will usually cut your calorie intake enough to begin reduction of body weight. But to attain an *ideal* body weight, it may be necessary to *plan* your calorie intake in order to control your reducing power pedal and to assure good health.

Low-calorie diets tend to be deficient in essential nutrients, so calories should not be reduced any lower than necessary, and only the most nutritious foods should be selected. Counting calories will enable you to divide your calorie intake among the basic energy nutrients as recommended in the U.S. Dietary Goals. The fewer calories your diet supplies the more important it is to budget your calories in a balanced diet.

When body weight is reduced gradually, at the rate of two or three pounds a week, it's more likely that weight loss will be permanent—and it can be accomplished without starvation or ill-ness. If you don't have much weight to lose and you want to lose only a pound or less a week, or if you want to avoid excessive weight loss, you can do so if you know how to control your reducing power pedal.

HOW TO CONTROL YOUR REDUCING POWER PEDAL
BY TAILORING YOUR CALORIE INTAKE

Generally, the average moderately active person must take in about 15 calories daily for each pound of body weight to maintain a desirable weight. Less active persons may need only 12 calories per pound of body weight, while persons who work hard might need as many as 18 calories per pound. When more calories are taken in than the body can use, the excess calories are stored as fat.

The average person burns from 2,500 to 3,000 calories a day. A sedentary person may need only 2,500 calories a day, while a person engaged in manual labor might need as many as 5,000 calories a day. Even if you don't do anything but sit all day, your body needs about 1,500 calories a day to carry on its basic functions. Respiration, digestion, heart action, and body metabolism, for example, burn calories. Such basic requirements are measured as the Basal Metabolic Rate (BMR). The average man's BMR consumes about 1,650 calories, while a woman's basic body functions consume about 1,350 calories. Since the basal metabolic rate declines with age, you'll need fewer calories as you grow older.

How to Burn Calories 24 Hours a Day

Although it is the consensus of experts that body conditioning cannot affect the basal metabolic rate, I have always felt that the more you exercise your muscles the more readily your body disposes of excess calories. It seems logical to me, for example, that the metabolic activity of well-toned muscles (which must repair or grow as a result of regular exercise) would burn calories 24 hours a day, even during rest. We know for certain that muscle tissue is more active metabolically than fat which is almost entirely inactive. This may explain why some people who exercise only 15 or 20 minutes every other day seem to be able to take in more calories than they burn in actual physical activity and still not gain weight.

I keep my muscles developed by lifting weights in a half-hour workout two or three times a week. Although I spend a total of only one to two hours a week exercising, I seem to be able to eat all I want without building up body fat. As long as my muscles are heavily developed, it seems that my calorie intake can exceed my calorie output with no problems whatsoever. A fat person, however, must make sure that calorie output exceeds calorie intake in order to burn off excess body fat. This must be done first by manipulating the diet. Exercise can then be used to *speed* weight loss.

Nutritious Calories vs. Empty Calories

Ideally, the calorie content of a reducing diet should not go below the basal metabolic requirement if adequate nutrients are to be obtained for basic body functions. This is one reason why it's never a good idea to go below 1,200 calories without medical supervision and why diets that supply less than 2,000 calories should be supplemented with vitamins and minerals. According to the National Academy of Sciences, "It is . . . difficult to assure nutritional adequacy of diets that are low in energy content (less than 1,800-2,000 kcal) unless fats, sugars, and alcohol are more rigidly restricted than is customary in most American households." (*Recommended Dietary Allowances*, 1974.)

Unfortunately, most Americans are eating so much fat and sugar and drinking so much alcohol that nutritional deficiencies are not uncommon in spite of a high calorie intake. With the average American drinking about 2.6 gallons of alcoholic beverages each year (supplying about 210 extra calories a day) and eating 125 pounds of fat and more than 100 pounds of sugar a year, it's no wonder that obesity is now the nation's No. 1 health and nutritional problem. (Alcohol supplies seven calories per gram, compared to nine calories per gram from fat and four calories per gram from carbohydrate.)

If you are really serious about reducing your body weight, you should not let sugar, fat, white flour, or alcohol displace nutritious foods in a low-calorie diet. The foods you eat must be high in nutrients and low in calories if you want to be healthy as well as slim.

Avoid Refined-Carbohydrate Calories

As I explained in Chapter 1, simply eliminating refined carbohydrates from the diet would result in weight loss for most people. When you are on a low-calorie reducing diet, it's absolutely essential that refined carbohydrates be replaced by natural carbohydrates. Most of us can tolerate the 10 percent energy intake from refined and processed sugars allowed by the U.S. Dietary Goals when maintaining body weight. But if you have developed a pancreatic sensitivity from excessive consumption of refined carbohydrates over a long period of time, including even a small amount of sugar and white flour in a reducing diet might make the diet less effective. One reason for this is that pancreatic sensitivity to sugar and other refined carbohydrates results in blood sugar fluctuations that force storage of blood sugar as fat, even on a low-calorie diet. You'll learn more about this in my discussion of hypoglycemia in Chapter 7.

In the meantime, remember that while you should try to exclude refined carbohydrates from your diet, you should continue to eat *natural* carbohydrates, whether you're counting calories or not.

HOW TO FIGURE CALORIE REQUIREMENT
ACCORDING TO BODY WEIGHT

Before you can cut your calorie intake down to a safe and effective level, you'll have to find out how many calories you should be taking in to weigh what you *should* weigh. You can use the height-weight chart in this chapter to roughly determine your ideal weight as based on *average* weights (Tables 3-1, 3-2). Or, if you are a man, you may estimate your ideal weight simply by beginning with a base weight of 106 pounds and adding five pounds for each inch over five feet of height. If you are a woman, begin with a base weight of 100 pounds and add five pounds for each inch of height over five feet. For each inch *under* five feet, you *subtract* five pounds.

Once you have estimated your ideal weight, you can estimate the number of calories you need to maintain that weight simply by multiplying calories per pound, depending upon how active you are.

WEIGHT CHART FOR MEN

Height (Nude)	Small Frame	Medium Frame	Large Frame	Average
5'2"	112-120	118-129	126-141	123
3"	115-123	121-133	129-144	127
4"	118-126	124-136	132-148	130
5"	121-129	127-139	135-152	133
6"	124-133	130-143	138-156	136
7"	128-137	134-147	142-161	140
8"	132-141	138-152	147-166	145
9"	136-145	142-156	151-170	149
10"	140-150	146-160	155-174	153
11"	144-154	150-165	159-179	158
6' 0"	148-158	154-170	164-184	162
1"	152-162	158-175	168-189	166
2"	156-167	162-180	173-194	171
3"	160-171	167-185	178-199	176
4"	164-175	172-190	182-204	181

Table 3-1

WEIGHT CHART FOR WOMEN

Height (Nude)	Small Frame	Medium Frame	Large Frame	Average
4'10"	92- 98	96-107	104-119	102
11"	94-101	98-110	106-122	104
5' 0"	96-104	101-113	109-125	107
1"	99-107	104-116	112-128	110
2"	102-110	107-119	115-131	113
3"	105-113	110-122	118-134	116
4"	108-116	113-126	121-138	120
5"	111-119	116-130	125-142	123
6"	114-123	120-135	129-146	128
7"	118-127	124-139	133-150	132
8"	122-131	128-143	137-154	136
9"	126-135	132-147	141-158	140
10"	130-140	136-151	145-163	144
11"	134-144	140-155	149-168	148
6' 0"	138-148	144-159	153-173	152

Table 3-2

A Formula for Calculating Calorie Requirement and Weight Loss

Assuming that you are an average moderately active person, you need about 15 calories for each pound of body weight to maintain your ideal weight, that is, what you *should* weigh. Calories in excess of that amount are stored as fat. Obviously, in order to lose weight, you would have to take in *fewer* calories than you would need to maintain your ideal weight. This would force your body to burn stored fat in partially meeting your energy needs. A 150-pound person, for example, would have to take in 2,250 calories a day to continue weighing 150 pounds (150 pounds × 15 calories = 2,250 calories). A 200-pound person who *should* weigh 150 pounds would have to take in *less* than 2,250 calories a day in order to lose weight. Since each pound of body fat contains about 3,500 calories, calorie intake would have to be reduced 500 calories a day (cut to 1,750) to lose *one pound* of fat a week. (A 500-calorie deficit multiplied by seven days equals 3,500 calories or one pound of fat.)

To lose *two pounds* of fat a week in reaching an ideal weight of 150 pounds, you'd have to limit your calorie intake to 1,250 calories a day, 1,000 fewer calories than needed to maintain a body weight of 150 pounds.

Remember that calorie requirements are figured according to what you *should* weigh. Be sure to estimate your ideal weight and the number of calories needed to maintain that weight before attempting to cut your calorie intake to lose weight. It's important that you have control of your reducing power pedal if you are to reduce your body weight safely and permanently.

Note: If you have only a few pounds to lose above your projected ideal weight, you may have to keep weight loss down to a pound or less a week in order to keep your calorie intake above 1,200 calories. For example, if you weigh 145 pounds and you need to lose only 10 pounds, you should not cut your calorie intake more than 500 calories a day. This will result in loss of one pound a week and allow you to consume 1,525 calories a day. Then, when your weight is down to 135 pounds, you can increase your energy intake to 2,025 calories a day in order to *maintain* that weight.

Burn Calories and Speed Weight Loss with Exercise

In addition to a dietary deficit of 1,000 calories a day for a weight loss of two pounds of fat a week, you can burn another 450 calories or more a day for an additional loss of a pound or more of body fat a week simply by being very active rather than moderately active. Of course, the more exercise you take the more calories you burn and the more fat you can lose on a controlled diet. How much you exercise is up to you. If you want to lose more than three pounds of fat a week on an adequate diet, you *should* exercise. Unless you participate in strenuous athletics, you should not expect to burn off more than two or three pounds of fat a week as a result of the exercise itself. *Combining* an adequate diet with a little regular exercise, however, can add up to a loss of five or six pounds of fat a week.

When your body weight reaches a predetermined weight goal, you must *increase* your calorie intake in order to maintain that weight. To maintain a weight of 150 pounds with moderate physical activity, for example, energy intake must be increased to 2,250 calories a day to prevent further weight loss (150 pounds × 15 calories = 2,250 calories). Remember that all calories should come from energy nutrients supplied by fresh, natural foods.

A QUICK REVIEW

After you have figured your calorie requirement, you should not forget to balance your diet by dividing your calorie intake among the basic energy nutrients—carbohydrate, protein, and fat—as suggested in Chapter 2. A 2,000 calorie reducing diet, for example, with 48 percent of calories coming from natural carbohydrate, 22 percent of calories coming from protein, and 30 percent of calories coming from fat, should supply about 960 carbohydrate calories, 440 protein calories, and 600 fat calories.

Since one gram of carbohydrate supplies four calories, 960 carbohydrate calories would equal *240 grams of carbohydrate.* One gram of protein supplies four calories, requiring *110 grams of protein* to provide 440 calories. Fat supplies nine calories per gram, so only *60 grams of fat* would be needed to supply 600 calories.

You can translate these gram figures into food servings by consulting the Table of Nutritive Values in Chapter 12.

Keep Carbohydrate High and Fat Low

You know from reading Chapter 2 that in the case of low-calorie diets (2,000 calories or less) I recommend that carbohydrate intake be limited to 48 percent of the energy requirement so that protein intake can be raised to 22 percent of the energy requirement to assure adequate protein. You should always make sure that you are getting *at least* 60 grams of protein (or about one gram of protein for each 2.2 pounds of ideal weight) and *more* than 100 grams of natural carbohydrate. Fat should *never* go above 30 percent of your energy intake.

On a higher-calorie maintenance diet (above 2,000 calorie), 58 *percent* of energy intake should come from natural carbohydrate, with 12 percent of calories coming from protein and 30 percent or less from fat.

Remember: Never go below 1,200 calories except when supervised by a physician. Always take a vitamin-and-mineral supplement when your diet supplies less than 2,000 calories. And make sure that you eat only fresh, natural foods.

Stick to the Basic Food Groups

If you select your foods properly from the basic four or seven food groups, you won't have to worry too much about measuring your energy nutrients too closely. A low-fat diet that supplies a moderate amount of protein with generous amounts of such natural carbohydrates as vegetables, fruits, and whole-grain products will usually add up to a balanced reducing diet. The modern dietary approach of dividing energy intake among all three energy nutrients (carbohydrate, protein, and fat) with emphasis on natural carbohydrate lends support to the old idea of spreading food selections over the seven basic food groups.

Gauging Calorie Intake by Weight Loss

Many people succeed in losing weight simply by eating a little less than usual. If you are presently *gaining* weight, however, you may be eating so much that you'll have to eat much less than you normally eat to force your body to burn stored fat. Cutting back only a little may help keep you from getting fatter but may not result in *loss* of weight. If you don't count calories to assure weight loss, just keep cutting back on your food intake until your scales begin to show a weight loss. But be sure to keep your diet balanced with food selections from all the basic food groups. While it's all right to cut down on the amount of food you eat, you should not eliminate any of the basic foods.

Don't weigh more often than once a week. Your body may be reluctant to release the water left over from combustion of fat, and it may release more water at one time than another. Weighing yourself every day may prove to be discouraging because of temporary retention of water. Your weight may even *increase* from one day to another, but it will ultimately *decrease* when leftover water is finally released.

Water retention might also be a problem when you're counting calories. If you're sure that your calorie intake is below that needed to maintain your ideal weight, and you're eating properly, stick with your diet and you'll eventually begin to shed excess body fat.

Average Results for Average People

The average person loses two to four pounds a week on a macro-nutrient diet. Some lose more and some less. A few persons will lose as much as seven pounds a week. If you lose only one or two pounds a week, don't despair. Studies have shown that persons who lose weight slowly are less likely to gain it back. Also, slower weight loss gives the skin time to retract so that it does not sag. Even if you lose only a pound or two a week, you'll eventually lose all of your excess body fat. Furthermore, you might look better than someone who loses more rapidly.

Remember that the rate of weight loss generally decreases as your body weight lessens. For this reason, you should not count on losing the same amount of weight week after week on the same diet.

Duncan V. experienced average weight loss on a macro-nutrient diet. After a loss of 14 pounds in six weeks, a little more than two pounds a week, he was one third of the way toward his weight goal. "I have plenty of energy, I feel good, and I'm not hungry," Duncan observed. "So why lose weight any faster?" I had no doubt that Duncan would eventually reach his weight goal.

Marguerite E. lost only about a pound and a half a week on her diet. But she lost a total of 65 pounds in 11 months. "This is the best diet ever," Marguerite insisted. "My skin is tight, my complexion is good, and I've had plenty of time to alter my clothes. I wouldn't consider going on any other diet."

WHY DIETING RESULTS VARY

There are many variables in dieting for weight loss. It's practically impossible to figure the exact number of calories supplied by a variety of foods. Also, since your physical activity may vary from day to day, you have no way of measuring your energy expenditure accurately. Dieting to lose weight is, at best, a procedure that requires *approximate* measurements. So don't worry about trying to figure your calorie intake and output down to the last calorie. No matter how closely you count your calories, you'll always be off a few hundred calories one way or the other. But if you make a reasonable effort at dieting and stay within a general range, you'll succeed in your effort and you'll eventually reach your weight goal.

Monitor Your Weight

Everyone's calorie needs may vary, even when height and weight are the same. You may have to monitor your weight and your actual food intake over a period of time before you can determine exactly how many calories you may take in or how much food you may eat to lose or maintain body weight. Obviously, dieting is not an exact science when it comes to the individual's needs. So don't follow someone else's diet. Apply what you learn from reading this book and then develop your own diet. You can determine from experience what is best for you.

Remember that you should not expect weight loss to conform exactly to your calorie computations. How your body gets rid of the water left over from the combustion of fat will have something to do with the rate and regularity of measurable weight loss. The fatter you are the more calories you'll burn just carrying the fat around. This is one reason why a heavier person may lose more weight faster than a lighter person following the same diet.

Anyone who has worked with reducing diets has observed the wide-ranging effects of such diets. Two people on the same diet rarely lose the same amount of weight. Erskin C., for example, had difficulty meeting the expected weight loss of two pounds a week on a 1,200 calorie diet. Arlene T., however, lost 5½ pounds the first week on the same diet and then lost an average of four pounds a week thereafter, losing a total of 33 pounds the first two months. Arlene had to *increase* her calorie intake on a maintenance diet after only three months of dieting. Erskin, on the other hand, had to plug along for several months before he finally reached his weight goal. Since Arlene was a hard-working housewife and Erskin a sedentary accountant, Arlene was probably burning more calories, and her well-toned muscles were probably disposing of calories 24 hours a day.

If you persist in eating properly, you'll eventually burn off excess body fat, just as Erskin did. Don't get impatient and starve yourself by going below 1,200 calories. It would be better to change food selections or take a little exercise. But whatever you do, be sure to continue dividing your energy intake among the various energy nutrients as instructed so that weight loss will be healthful and permanent.

DRINK PLENTY OF WATER AND REDUCE
YOUR SALT INTAKE

If you are healthy, drinking water will *not* result in a gain in body weight. In fact, it's a good idea to drink plenty of water to aid your kidneys in eliminating uric acid and other by-products of weight reduction. But you should keep your salt intake to a minimum, since too much salt will force retention of water. The U.S. Dietary Goals have advised us to limit our intake of table salt to about five grams (one teaspoon) a day. Since salt (sodium chloride) is about 40 percent sodium, five grams (5,000 milligrams) of salt supply about 2,000 milligrams of sodium. This is actually more sodium than the body needs—and it's the sodium in salt that does the damage.

Too much sodium in the diet upsets the balance of sodium and potassium in the blood, affecting the flow of water through tissue cells, thus upsetting the balance of water in the body. Water retention won't contribute to the formation of fat, but it can contribute to swollen ankles, eye bags, and high blood pressure. Ingestion of an excessive amount of sodium over a long period of time might also contribute to the development of hardened arteries. And once the body has been damaged, anything can happen.

Fortunately, a healthy body will usually eliminate moderate excesses of dietary sodium through urine and perspiration. This elimination is aided by drinking water. This is one reason why eating salty foods makes you thirsty. When you are on a reducing diet, it's best to consume as little table salt as possible, but you should still drink plenty of water. In fact, a glass of water before each meal will help reduce your appetite by filling your stomach.

Avoid Sodium Additives

Your body needs only about one fourth of a gram (250 milli-grams) of sodium for good health. So you can get all the sodium you need from natural foods. Unless you are sweating profusely for long periods of time in labor or athletics and you lose more than four quarts of water, you don't need extra salt. Iodized table salt helps to prevent iodine deficiency, but if you include seafood in your diet as you should, you'll get adequate iodine. Except for an occasional taste treat or for medical reasons, therefore, you should avoid add-ing salt to your diet.

Processed foods are often rich in sodium in the form of salt, additives, or preservatives, such as monosodium glutamate and sodium nitrate. Furthermore, processing a food may result in loss of potassium, further upsetting the balance between sodium and potassium. If you want to prevent imbalances that force your body to retain the water released in the combustion of fats and carbohy-drates, *stick to natural foods and avoid the salt shaker.* You'll get better results on your reducing diet and you'll be able to measure the effects of your calorie counting more accurately.

A Zero-Calorie Beverage!

Water does not contain calories. You can drink all the water you want—and the more the better. Try to drink at least six glasses a day. "Everytime I pass a sink," says actor Joseph Campanella, "I'll drink half a glass of water—not a full glass but *half* a glass. I drink a total of eight to 10 glasses of water a day."

Although water does not contain calories, it does contain min-erals, and it may be high in sodium. Call your local water depart-ment and ask for an analysis of the drinking water. If the sodium content of the water is unusually high (more than 100 milligrams per liter), you might want to get your drinking water elsewhere if you suffer from hypertension or heart trouble. Ideally, drinking water should probably not contain more than 20 milligrams of sodium per liter. (A liter is a little more than a quart.) Water softeners greatly increase the sodium content of water. Try to avoid drinking artificially softened water.

I do not recommend drinking distilled water. When water is distilled, all the minerals are left behind, and you *need* the minerals supplied by water. Some scientists have observed, for example, that in areas where the drinking water is high in magnesium there is a lower incidence of sudden death from heart failure. When you are unable to drink local water because of a high sodium content, it would be better to drink bottled mineral water than to drink distilled water.

Natural Carbohydrates Are Rich in Water

Foods also supply water. And when a food's water content is high, chances are the food is low in calories. Natural carbohydrates such as fresh fruits and vegetables contain more water than anything else. This is one reason why they are useful diet foods. Most fruits and vegetables, for example, contain from 70 to 95 percent water. Meats, on the other hand, contain from 40 to 75 percent water, depending upon their fat content. Whole-grain products are only eight to 20 percent water, but they are rich in fiber—and you need fiber to hold water in your intestinal tract.

Your Body Is Over Half Water

From one half to three fourths (about 60 percent) of your body weight is water, depending upon your age and the amount of body fat you have. Muscle tissue is rich in water while fat tissue contains very little water. A lean body, therefore, contains a greater percentage of water than a fat body. (Ideally, a man's body is about 18 percent fat, while a woman's body is about 22 percent fat.)

When you are reducing your body weight, it's the excess *fat* you want to lose and not water. In fact, water is so essential in the body's metabolic functions that you cannot afford to lose more than 10 percent of your body water. This is one reason why the water loss on low-carbohydrate diets is so dangerous.

Your body normally loses about six percent of its water (a pint or two) each day through urine, perspiration, bowel movements, and respiration. This water is easily replaced by proper eating and drinking habits. Oxidation of carbohydrate, protein, and fat in the body produces water that is retained by the body if the diet is properly balanced. If the diet is deficient in carbohydrate, forcing the body to burn an excessive amount of fat for energy, large amounts of water are lost in flushing ketones and other waste products from the body. So it's just as important to include natural carbohydrates in a balanced diet as it is to drink plenty of water if you want to protect your health and reduce your body weight safely and permanently.

WHAT ABOUT FASTING?

It's never a good idea to restrict calorie intake with total fasting—at least not for longer than a day or two. When your body's store of glycogen is depleted (after one to three days of fasting) and carbohydrate is no longer available to supply glucose and replenish glycogen stores, your body begins to burn muscle protein along with fat. The muscle protein is converted to glucose to provide your brain with fuel, and body fat is broken down to feed other body cells. Ketones, the toxic residue left over when fat is burned in the absence of carbohydrate, literally overload your kidneys and dehydrate your body. The production of ketones from excessive burning of fat also kills your appetite, allowing your body to feed upon itself without any sense of hunger. This means that you can starve yourself to death without a desire for food.

Although your body can manufacture carbohydrate (glucose) from protein, you must include some preformed carbohydrate in your diet to prevent ketosis, excessive breakdown of body protein, loss of sodium and other important minerals, and to prevent dehydration from excessive loss of body water. According to the National Research Council, "Fifty to one hundred grams of digestible carbohydrate a day will offset the undesirable metabolic responses associated with high fat diets and fasting."

You Can Burn More Fat by Eating than by Fasting!

In prolonged fasting, nutritional deficiencies and loss of such water-soluble minerals as sodium, potassium, and calcium depress the heart rate and disturb metabolic functions. Without the vitamins and minerals that must be supplied *daily* in a balanced diet, the body's resistance to disease is lowered. It's all right to fast for a day or two occasionally. But remember that prolonged fasting is simply starvation. And when the body is forced to feed entirely upon itself, health may be permanently impaired. Many people on fasting diets report hair loss as well as an irregular heart rate, a fall in blood pressure, anemia, gouty arthritis, fatigue, nausea, headache, and other side effects. Also, only 15 percent of lost tissue may be fat, with muscle wasting accounting for most of the weight loss.

Actually, you can lose more body fat by eating than by fasting! Studies show, for example, that *70 percent of weight loss on a low-calorie diet is fat compared to only 15 percent on a fasting diet.* Less fat is burned on a fasting diet because the body is forced to convert muscle protein to glucose to feed the nervous system. Since body fat cannot be converted to glucose, your own muscles must supply the glucose normally provided by the carbohydrate in your diet. Obviously, you must include some natural carbohydrate in your reducing diet if you are to control your fat-burner throttle so that you burn fat instead of muscle. You learned in Chapter 2 that 48 to 58 percent of your energy should come from carbohydrate. So you already know that fasting is not the answer. You must *eat* to lose body fat safely. Weight loss may be a little slower, but you'll lose *fat* instead of muscle and water.

The Case of William R.

William R. had a habit of fasting periodically in an attempt to shed body fat that had accumulated from months of unrestricted eating. "I'd rather fast occasionally than go on a long diet," William explained, "so that I can eat what I want most of the time." William's fasting did show a weight loss on the scales, but much of the weight loss was muscle and water. And just as soon as he started eating again, the body water and the muscle protein were quickly replaced. Fat continued to accumulate from overeating. The result was that at the end of each year William weighed a little more than the year before. When he suffered a heart attack, he finally expressed a desire to change his eating habits. I recommended my macro-nutrient diet.

"I lost 70 pounds in 12 months," William later reported ecstatically. "And I did it without fasting. In fact, I did it by eating! Best of all, my blood fat is normal for the first time in years. My doctor told me that the blood vessels around my heart are no longer clogged. I'm feeling fine. If I can lose weight safely on a macro-nutrient diet, anyone can!"

Low-Carbohydrate Diets Have Fasting Effects

It's absolutely essential that you eat something each day and that your diet include natural carbohydrate as well as protein. If you're overweight, you must also make sure that you take in fewer calories each day than your body burns. You can then lose two or three pounds a week safely and surely without fasting. You'll have full control of your reducing power pedal.

Most fasting diets result in a loss of a pound or more of body weight daily. About 65 percent of this weight loss may be muscle tissue, however, and all weight loss over one pound may be mostly water. You have to *burn* off fat to get rid of it—and a pound of fat supplies 3,500 calories. To create a 3,500-calorie deficit to burn off a pound of fat a day, you'd have to burn 2,000 calories or more daily in addition to the 1,500 consumed by your basal metabolism. This would be difficult to do without total fasting or without exercising strenuously. Since fasting results in nutritional deficiencies that preclude exercise, the only safe way to lose weight is to lose slowly on a good diet that allows a dietary deficit of only 1,000 or so calories a day. You may then combine exercise with the diet for faster weight loss.

Any diet that restricts or excludes carbohydrate is a fasting diet and can have many of the effects of total fasting. It may, in fact, be just about as harmful to go on a zero-carbohydrate diet as to eat nothing at all. If you do restrict your carbohydrate intake for some reason, you should drink planty of water to aid your kidneys in flushing out ketones and uric acid and to combat dehydration. But you shouldn't stay on such a diet for more than a few days.

COUNT DOWN ON BODY FAT

It's usually not too hard to determine when you have lost enough weight. A quick look in the mirror will tell the story. If you can pinch up more than one inch of fat on your abdomen or on the back of your upper arm, you still have too much fat. If you pinch up less than half an inch of fat, you're too thin. It may be difficult to determine when you have reached your ideal weight, even with the use of scales. When you are pleased with your physical appearance, it's not likely that you need to lose any more weight. It's a good idea, however, to determine beforehand what the average ideal weight is for someone of your height and frame. You can do this simply by consulting the height-weight chart in this chapter. When you reach your weight goal and you cannot pinch up more than one inch of fat on your abdomen, you may then increase your calorie intake and go on a maintenance diet.

Occasionally, weight loss becomes such an obsession that dieting becomes an emotional disease (anorexia nervosa) that leads to starvation. When this happens, healthful body fat is lost along with precious muscle protein. If you feel that you should weigh much less than the ideal weight given for your height and frame, see your doctor and ask him if he thinks you are too fat. A disinterested professional person will be more objective than you in evaluating your appearance.

Generally if you weigh 10 percent more than the desirable weight given on a standard height-weight chart, you may be overweight. If you are 20 percent heavier than you should be, you might be *obese*. Of course, desirable weights for individuals will vary, depending upon bone size and muscle bulk. Remember that height-weight charts represent *average* weights. A body builder or an athlete might not be represented on a weight chart. Your best weight is the weight at which you look best and function best, regardless of what the charts say.

A Little Fat Can Be Attractive!

Carolee A. lost 23 pounds in three months on a macronutrient diet. "I'm still 10 pounds overweight according to the weight chart," Carolee noted, "but I don't really believe I should lose any more weight." I agreed. Carolee was slightly pudgy, but she looked great. Her body lines were full but firm, and she was certainly physically appealing. As long as she felt good about herself and was pleased with the way she looked, it wasn't necessary for her to lose more weight just to meet someone else's standard.

You, too, might prefer to be a little heavier than the recommended weight for someone of your height and frame. Some persons do look better with a little extra body fat. It could be that you do, too. Just be honest with yourself—and then use your best judgment.

MORE EXAMPLES OF SUCCESSFUL, BENEFICIAL
WEIGHT LOSS

Many benefits accompany successful weight loss. Here are a few more examples of persons who were able to improve their lives by shedding excess body fat on a macro-nutrient diet.

Aubrey R. reduced his wastline from 42 inches to 35 inches when he went on a macro-nutrient diet to remove 21 pounds of fat from his body. "I can sit more comfortably and breathe better since I got rid of that roll of fat around my waist," Aubrey reported happily, "but what I appreciate most of all is the improvement in my golf score!"

Ormond L. was a lead guitarist and vocalist in a popular band. When he overheard someone in the audience refer to him as "that fatso musician," he decided to go on a macro-nutrient type of diet. He lost 53 pounds in 17 weeks. "I knew my diet was succeeding," Ormond confided, "when I started getting a lot more attention from the girls who came to hear us play."

Forty-four-year-old Minnie D. was having sexual problems that she attributed to an overabundance of body fat. After losing 43 pounds of fat on a macro-nutrient diet, her sex life improved tremendously. "I now feel more like having sex," Minnie reported, "and my husband is more turned on than ever before. Physical appearance obviously has a lot to do with sexual performance."

Jackson O. lost his job when it became apparent that excess body fat was hindering his performance as an electrician. Drawing upon his instinct for survival, he persisted with macro-nutrient dieting until he lost more than 150 pounds of fat! "Getting fired for being too fat was the best thing that ever happened to me," Jackson stated emphatically. "I've been going so strong since reducing my body weight that I now have my own business. And no one doubts that I can do the job."

Rima G. spent most of her evenings at home alone because she was obese. "When I hear someone say that I have a nice face and good personality, I know they're looking at my fat," she wailed. Rima employed the principles of macro-nutrient dieting to make sure that she shed her fat safely and permanently. She got rid of 100 pounds of fat in seven months! "I know from experience that fat women don't have as much fun as other women," Rima confided, "because I'm having more fun and more dates now than I ever had before. I didn't dare go disco dancing when I was fat. Now I go a couple of times a week—and I have several boy friends."

All of these stories are typical of persons who shed excess body fat on a macro-nutrient type of diet. Anyone who transforms his or her body from bulging obesity to lithe leanness can tell a similar story. Every phase of life can be affected by body weight. Your health, your happiness, your future, and your longevity could very well depend upon what you do to control your body weight. This book, therefore, might be the most important book you'll ever read.

SUMMARY

1. *Consult the height-weight chart in this chapter to determine what the average ideal weight is for a person with your frame.*
2. *In order to maintain an ideal weight, the average moderately active person must take in about 15 calories per pound of body weight.*
3. *To lose two pounds a week, you must take in 1,000 fewer calories a day than needed to maintain your ideal weight.*
4. *When your weight goal is reached, calorie intake should be increased to maintain that weight.*
5. *Since calorie counting is not always accurate, you may have to monitor your weight and your food intake over a period of time to learn how to eat to control your body weight.*
6. *Because a pound of fat contains 3,500 calories, it's difficult to eat properly and lose more than two or three pounds of body fat a week without exercising.*
7. *When you are on a reducing diet, it's important to drink plenty of water and reduce your salt intake to a minimum.*
8. *Loss of more than one pound of body weight a day without the help of exercise might mean excessive loss of body water or muscle protein as a result of a bad diet.*
9. *If you can pinch up more than one inch of fat on your abdomen or on the back of your upper arm, you may have too much fat, regardless of what the scales say.*
10. *Fasting longer than a day or two depletes glycogen stores and forces the body to convert muscle protein to glucose in order to provide fuel for the nervous system.*

4

How to Get the Nutrients
You Need from Delicious
Macro-Nutrient Foods

The new U.S. Dietary Goals, as you have learned, tell you how to distribute your energy intake among the various energy nutrients so that you increase your intake of natural carbohydrate and decrease your intake of sugar, salt, and fat. The purpose of these goals is to encourage Americans to make greater use of dietary measures in preventing disease. The amount of food you eat and the number of calories you take in, however, must be tailored to your needs. Once you learn how to balance the energy nutrients in your diet, you can adjust your calorie intake according to your body weight, as I have suggested in Chapters 2 and 3. But it's not enough to simply control your calorie intake by adjusting your servings of carbohydrate, protein, and fat. *You must make sure that you get all the vitamins and minerals you need for the best of health.* To do this, you must select and prepare your foods carefully.

What you learn in this chapter will help you be healthy as well as slim. So be sure to follow its guidelines in developing your macro-nutrient diet.

"A macro-nutrient diet is not like other diets I've tried," observed Carlson T., who lost 30 pounds in eight weeks. "I was hardly even aware that I was on a diet. I had plenty to eat. I ate only *fresh* foods—and they were absolutely delicious. I'm now on a macro-nutrient maintenance diet, and it's a snap. The only difference is that I'm eating more and enjoying it more. My weight is staying the same."

Leona S. lost 35 pounds in 12 weeks. "I couldn't believe it," Leona said, "until I switched from a size 18 dress to a junior 10! The diet was a pleasure. The results were fantastic. I'd recommend a macro-nutrient diet for anyone, even persons who love to eat. Once you learn how to select and prepare foods, dieting is simple."

FOOD PREPARATION IS IMPORTANT

If you eat fresh, natural foods in a balanced diet as recommended in the opening chapters of this book, you'll have half the battle won in your effort to eat properly. How you *prepare* some of the foods you eat, however, can be a deciding factor in meeting your nutritional requirements. You already know that reducing diets should never go below 1,200 calories and that diets that supply fewer than 2,000 calories should be supplemented with vitamins and minerals. But even when you take supplements, you must do everything you can to make sure that the foods you eat retain as many of their nutrients as possible. One reason for this is that natural foods may contain undiscovered nutrients that are as essential for good health as the 50 or more nutrients (13 essential vitamins and 15 essential minerals) we already know about. You cannot depend entirely upon bottled supplements for good health. It's absolutely essential that you do everything you can to conserve nutrients in the foods you eat, especially when you are eating a small amount of food on a low-calorie diet.

ADJUSTING TO FOOD PROBLEMS

You'll learn in this chapter how to prepare foods so that they are nutritious as well as tasty. You'll also learn how to handle special food problems that might affect your intake of nutrients. If you cannot tolerate the lactose (sugar) in milk, for example, you can switch to *fermented* milk products in which lactose has been converted to lactic acid. Persons who are allergic to the gluten in wheat, rye, oats, and barley will have to avoid all grains except corn and rice. Vegetarians who refuse to eat the flesh of our fellow creatures can get the protein and the Vitamin B12 they need from other foods. Combinations of rice and beans, for example, can supply needed protein. Milk products can supply Vitamin B12 as well as protein.

When you cannot eat certain basic foods for some reason, you'll have to learn how to make special adjustments in your diet in order to get all the essential nutrients. You'll learn more about how to do this when you read Chapter 5. In the meantime, since food selections should be made from *all* the basic food groups whenever possible, let's start with the milk group in learning how to maximize nutrients while minimizing calories. Remember that on a reducing diet *you must get more nutrients from a smaller amount of food.* So it's important to make sure that you eat nutritious, low-calorie foods that have been *properly prepared.*

HOW TO GET YOUR SHARE OF NUTRIENTS
FROM THE MILK GROUP

Nutritionists recommend that the average adult include two or more cups of milk (or its equivalent in milk products) in the diet each day to assure an adequate intake of calcium. On a macro-nutrient slimming diet, you'll be consuming *skim* milk and its products. Removing fat from milk removes its Vitamin A but has no effect on its calcium, riboflavin, Vitamin B12, and protein content. Since fat is high in calories and may contribute to the development of heart disease, overweight, and other problems in adults, you can afford to sacrifice the Vitamin A of whole milk for less fat and fewer calories. If your diet is properly balanced, you'll get the Vitamin A you need from liver, eggs, dark green and yellow vegetables and fruits, fortified skim milk and its products, and other foods.

Cutting the Fat from Milk

Skim milk provides only a little more than half the number of calories found in whole milk. A cup of *whole milk*, for example, which is about 3.5 percent fat, contains nine grams of fat and 160 calories. *Skim milk* has only a trace of fat with about 90 calories per cup. *Low-fat milk* is only partially skimmed and may be from one percent to two percent fat. One cup of two percent low-fat milk contains about five grams of fat and 145 calories. Obviously, if you drink a lot of milk, you'll get less fat and fewer calories from skim milk than from whole milk or low-fat milk.

Eliminating milk fat from your diet will enable you to operate your reducing power pedal much more effectively. This does not apply to children, however. The U.S. Dietary Goals recommend that young children consume *whole milk* and its products. It is the consensus of experts that growing children should *not* be deprived of the calories and the fat-soluble nutrients supplied by whole milk.

Persons who enjoy buttermilk should ask for the cultured variety made from skim milk. One cup of low-fat buttermilk contains only 90 calories and a trace of fat.

When buying milk products, select low-fat products made from skim milk. Low-fat yogurt and uncreamed cottage cheese, for example, contain all the nutrients of skim milk minus milk sugar.

Coping with Lactose Intolerance

Many adults have trouble digesting the lactose (sugar) in fresh milk. The intestinal tract normally produces an enzyme called lactase which breaks down lactose (into glucose and galactose) so that it can be absorbed. After the age of four, however, many of us are no longer able to digest milk sugar because of failure of the intestinal tract to produce lactase. This results in flatulence, stomach cramps, diarrhea, and other digestive symptoms when milk is consumed. If you have this problem, don't despair. You don't have to deprive yourself of the nutrients supplied by milk simply because you are intolerant of lactose. You can now purchase the lactase enzyme in tablet form. Taking these tablets with milk will enable you to digest milk normally.

Solve Your Problem with Fermented Milk Products

If you cannot digest lactose (and lactase tablets are not available to you), all you have to do is select the *fermented* variety of milk and its products. When milk is fermented with a bacterial culture, the lactose is converted to lactic acid. Buttermilk, cottage cheese, yogurt, farmer's cheese, and pot cheese, for example, are fermented milk products. All of these products convey the benefits of milk without the milk sugar. Yogurt and cultured buttermilk offer the additional benefit of providing the intestinal tract with healthful, friendly bacteria that aid digestion and produce an acid environment that inhibits the growth of unfriendly bacteria.

Try to make sure that the yogurt or buttermilk you consume contains *live* bacteria. Many commercial yogurts, especially frozen yogurts, have been cooked and therefore contain *dead* bacteria. When such yogurts have been sweetened with sugar or preserves, they're no better than ice cream. Read labels carefully. When you are on a reducing diet, you don't need sweetened yogurts that may be high in calories. Plain yogurt served with fresh fruit or with sliced raw vegetables is best. A chilled mixture of plain yogurt and cultured buttermilk makes a great low-calorie "sour cream" dressing for a baked potato.

Create Your Own Living Yogurt

You can make sure that the yogurt you eat is alive by making your own. You can also control the fermentation to make the yogurt sweet or tart to suit your taste. And you can add milk powder to give the yogurt more firmness. You should, of course, use skim milk and nonfat milk powders to make a low-calorie yogurt.

You can purchase a yogurt-making kit in most health food stores where you can get supplies along with instructions. Lactobacillus bulgaricus in combination with other bacteria is the most commonly used culture. Once you have a batch of live yogurt on hand, you can use a small amount of the yogurt as a starter for making a new supply. It might be a good idea to boil milk before using it to make yogurt, that is, before adding the culture. This will kill the bacteria normally found in milk so that the yogurt bacteria will be free to grow. While making yogurt, however, the temperature of the milk must not go above 120 degrees Fahrenheit. You'll learn more in the next chapter about how to make yogurt.

Milk Products Supply Essential Calcium and Vitamin B12

Without milk or milk products in your diet, it might be difficult to get adequate calcium, riboflavin, and protein. So be sure to include at least two cups of milk (or its equivalent in milk products) in your diet every day. If you don't eat much meat, you'll need the Vitamin B12 as well as the protein supplied by milk. (Milk loses riboflavin when exposed to light. Keep your milk in light-proof containers in a dark place.)

Persons who cannot tolerate milk in any form can get calcium and protein from *soy milk*, a milk substitute made from soybeans. If you exclude cow's milk and its products from your diet, however, you'll have to depend upon other animal products for your Vitamin B_{12}.

Avoid Synthetic Dairy Products

Non-dairy creamers are synthetic products that may contain harmful additives as well as saturated fat. The "vegetable oil" used in synthetic cream, for example, is often coconut oil, which is highly saturated. Use skim milk instead of cream or non-dairy creamers in your coffee.

You should also avoid processed cheeses, since they often contain unnatural ingredients. Cheddar, Colby, Swiss, and other natural yellow cheeses made from whole milk are healthful, but they are high in fat and must be used sparingly in a reducing diet. Try to stick with the skim milk variety of cheese, such as *un-creamed cottage cheese*, until you get your weight down.

HOW TO GET MEAT NUTRIENTS WITHOUT FAT

In the meat group, it's usually recommended that you have two or more servings daily of beef, veal, pork, lamb, poultry, fish, or eggs, with dry beans and peas or nuts as alternate dishes. On a low-fat reducing diet, you should, of course, select lean cuts of meat and then cut away all visible fat. The meat may then be baked, broiled, or cooked in some other manner that will minimize fat content. This means no frying with oil and no cooking with batters. Fats cooked out of meats should be drained away and discarded.

Cheaper Meats Are Usually Leaner Meats

Cheaper, lower-grade meats usually contain less fat than "choice" or "prime" cuts of meat. "Good" grades of meat, for example, contain more muscle and less fat and are therefore tougher but more healthful. They also provide a better fuel for your reducing power pedal.

Tough meats can be tenderized by cooking them in the presence of moisture, as in boiling, stewing, or braising. When you boil meats, remember that the water-soluble B vitamins dissolve into the cooking water. You can chill the leftover water and then skim off the hard surface fat so that the water can be used as a sauce to pour over baked potatoes, dry meat, and other foods.

Substitutes for Meat Dishes

Generally, we eat meat to supply protein, B vitamins, and iron. Since red meats are rich in saturated fat and cholesterol, we are usually advised to eat more fish and poultry and less beef and pork. Cutting your intake of red meats, however, will reduce your intake of iron. This means that you'll have to get more iron from whole eggs, beans, fruits, and dark green leafy vegetables.

When you do use alternate dishes to replace the protein supplied by meat, you can substitute two eggs, a cup of dried beans, or four tablespoons of peanut butter for a three-ounce serving of meat. Eggs offer a complete protein, but peas, beans, and peanut butter are not complete. If your meal is balanced to include milk and whole-grain products, combining these foods with beans or peanut butter in the same meal will produce a complete protein. Since milk provides a complete protein, combining milk with whole-grain products and other sources of incomplete protein will actually *increase* the total amount of complete protein in your meal.

Soybeans Are Nearly Equal to Meat

Soybeans are rich in protein and iron and make an excellent substitute dish for meat. Iron is more easily absorbed from meat than from beans and other vegetables, but iron supplied by a variety of foods, including fish and poultry, should be adequate. Although soybeans do contain some fat, they contain more protein and less fat than most meats. The soybean in its natural state, for example, contains 40 percent protein compared to only 18 percent protein in meat. And because of their lower fat content, soybeans supply fewer calories than most meats. A cup of cooked soybeans contains the same amount of protein as a lamb chop but about 100 fewer calories!

You can mix textured soybeans with hamburger or meat loaf to produce a nutritious, low-calorie meat dish. Or you can purchase mixtures of ground meat and soybeans. You should, of course, use a low-fat ground meat such as ground round steak. Some ground meats contain more fat than protein. A quarter-pound hamburger, for example, might contain 32 grams of fat and only 27 grams of protein.

Although soybeans supply a complete protein, they are weak in a few of the essential amino acids, thus providing protein that is not equal in quality to that supplied by meat. For this reason, you should include wheat, corn, rice, or milk with meals that totally substitute soybeans for meat. This will assure higher quality protein. But remember that while soybeans can supply some of the iron and most of the protein you would normally get from red meat, you'll have to depend upon milk and other animal products for Vitamin B_{12}. (*Fermented* soy products, such as tempeh, supply some Vitamin B_{12}).

Warning: Raw soybeans may be poisonous, and they contain a substance that can interfere with absorption of Vitamins A and B_{12}. Always *cook* your soybeans—and make sure that they are well done. Properly cooked, soybeans supply some Vitamin A as well as calcium, phosphorus, iron, thiamine, and riboflavin. The lecithin supplied by soybeans contains choline and inositol which are believed to be useful in lowering blood cholesterol and improving the function of the nervous system.

Reducing the Fat in Peanut Butter

Peanut butter is rich in protein but, like most legumes, is weak in one or more of the essential amino acids. Luckily, grains are strong in the same amino acids that are weak in the peanut butter. You can make a complete, high-quality protein by combining peanut butter with whole-grain bread. Whenever possible, however, you should include milk or some other animal product in your meal when you substitute peanut butter for a meat dish.

Unfortunately, peanut butter is high in fat, so it should not be eaten in large quantities very often, especially when you are on a reducing diet. When you do eat peanut butter, it should be the natural variety in which the peanut oil rises to the top of the jar. You can then pour off the oil to reduce the total number of fat calories. Joyce DeWitt of TV's "Three's Company" places a freshly opened jar of natural peanut butter upside down in a bowl containing paper napkins and leaves it that way overnight to drain off excess oil.

Most of the peanut butter sold in grocery stores has been hydrogenated. This means that hydrogen has been added to *harden* peanut oil so that it won't spoil or rise to the top of the jar. This converts the oil to a saturated fat that may be as bad for your arteries as for your waistline. Such peanut butter usually also contains sugar, lard, and other fattening or harmful ingredients. You can purchase a fresh, natural peanut butter in any health food store. If you prefer, you can make your own peanut butter at home by putting lightly roasted peanuts into a blender.

Eggs Are a Superior Source of Protein

Egg white offers the best available high-quality protein, followed by milk, fish, cheese, and meat and poultry—in that order. Egg yolks, however, may have to be eaten sparingly because of their high cholesterol content. In a balanced diet in which a variety of foods can be depended upon for protein, you won't need to eat more than one whole egg a day. (Most doctors recommend no more than four eggs a week.)

The Vitamin A, Vitamin D, and other fat-soluble nutrients in egg yolk are especially helpful in a low-fat diet. Egg yolk is one of the few foods that naturally contain Vitamin D. The only vitamin missing in egg yolk is Vitamin C. So an egg—a *whole* egg—is a highly nutritious food. If you don't already have a high blood cholesterol, don't worry about the cholesterol content of egg yolk. Eating an egg or two a day will *not* raise your blood cholesterol if you are healthy. No one knows for sure what causes an abnormal elevation in blood cholesterol, but many nutritionists now maintain that moderate use of eggs is not a factor. Once your blood cholesterol is highly elevated, however, for whatever reason, you may then have to restrict consumption of egg yolk.

The best way to cook an egg to preserve its nutrients is to soft boil the egg in its shell. Or you may poach, scramble, or fry an egg as long as you do so without use of oil or excessive heat. You can use a special coated pan to fry an egg without oil. Try to avoid cooking an egg yolk until it is hard. Overcooking an egg destroys the lecithin and essential fatty acids that emulsify the cholesterol in the yolk. Raw eggs, on the other hand, contain avidin, a substance that prevents absorption of the B vitamin biotin. So while you should not overcook your eggs, you should not eat them raw, either.

Selecting a Low-Fat Meat

The leaner cuts of beef (such as veal, tenderloin, chuck steak, or roast), chicken or turkey without the skin, leg of lamb, and fresh fish are all low in fat. Your best bet for meeting your protein requirement on a reducing diet, however, is to eat *fish or poultry* that has been prepared without grease or oil. In addition to being low in fat, fish and poultry are largely unsaturated. And fish, like egg yolk, is one of the few available food sources of Vitamin D.

Poultry can be prepared in many ways, such as baking, broiling, stewing, barbecuing, and so on. Fish is probably best cooked by broiling, steaming, or poaching. It takes only a small amount of heat to cook fish adequately. When the flesh of fish changes from translucent to an opaque white, it is cooked enough. Properly cooked fish can be easily flaked with a fork. When overcooked, fish becomes dry and tough. For additional information on how to cook fish, see *Let's Cook Fish!*, available from the National Marine Fisheries Service, Washington, D.C. 20240.

BALANCE YOUR NUTRIENT INTAKE WITH
VEGETABLES AND FRUITS

Fruits and vegetables are good sources of natural carbohydrate, and they contain the fiber and the nutrients you need to balance your diet. Both fruits and vegetables are high in water and fiber and low in calories. But since vegetables generally contain fewer calories than fruits, vegetables should supply the greater portion of your carbohydrate intake, Remember that about 58 percent of your energy intake should be supplied by natural carbohydrate. When there is adequate carbohydrate in your reducing diet, your fat-burner throttle will burn *body fat* rather than muscle protein in producing fuel from a limited supply of energy nutrients. (For an explanation of how carbohydrate spares protein, read the material on fasting in Chapter 3.)

The Seven Basic Food Groups Favor Vegetables

The four basic food groups list vegetables and fruits in one group, asking you to consume four or more servings from that group daily. You are advised to select a dark green or a deep yellow vegetable at least every other day. Otherwise, you are allowed to substitute fruits for vegetables in most of your selections. Fruits may meet your nutritional requirements, but they may also supply a few extra calories. An orange, for example, supplies about 65 calories (with 66 milligrams of Vitamin C), while a tomato supplies only 25 calories (with 28 milligrams of Vitamin C). Since citrus fruits are generally the best available source of Vitamin C, they should be included in generous amounts in your diet. But *vegetables* should supply the greater part of your carbohydrate intake.

The seven basic food groups include vegetables in their first three groups, thus assuring a predominance of vegetables. I listed the seven basic food groups in Chapter 1, but here they are again: (1) green and yellow vegetables; (2) citrus fruit, tomatoes, and raw cabbage; (3) potatoes and other vegetables and fruits; (4) skim milk and its products; (5) lean meat, skinned poultry, fish, eggs, and dried peas and beans; (6) whole-grain bread, cereal, and flour; and (7) butter, margarine, and vegetable oil. If you eat something from each of these seven groups each day, chances are you'll eat more vegetables than fruits and you'll automatically balance your diet.

Note: In my version of the seven basic food groups, I recommend the low-fat, unprocessed variety of foods, whether you are on a reducing diet or not.

Fruits for Vitamin C, Vegetables for Vitamin A

Although both fruits and vegetables supply Vitamin A as well as Vitamin C, we eat fruits primarily for their Vitamin C. We depend more upon dark green and deep yellow vegetables for their Vitamin A. Since Vitamin C can be easily destroyed by heat or washed away by water, you should always eat your fruits *raw*. Vegetables lose most of their Vitamin C when they are cooked. Most of the vegetables you eat will be cooked to improve their taste, but very few vegetables must be cooked to be edible. Try to eat a variety of raw vegetables in a fresh, crisp salad every day.

Fortunately, the Vitamin A in vegetables is not destroyed by cooking. In fact, a small amount of cooking to soften the cellulose in vegetables will release a greater amount of Vitamin A for absorption by your body. This is why you should eat both raw *and* cooked vegetables—to increase your intake of both Vitamin C and Vitamin A.

Actually, vegetables supply *carotene,* a Vitamin A precursor that is converted to Vitamin A in your body. Preformed Vitamin A is found only in animal products and must be absorbed in the presence of fat. Unlike preformed Vitamin A, carotene is nontoxic. Excessive consumption of carotene from carrots or carrot juice might turn your skin yellow, but no physical harm will result. You don't need yellow skin any more than you need a Vitamin A overdose, however. So don't go overboard on the use of carrot juice as a beverage.

You can eat generous amounts of cooked vegetables that are prepared without grease or oil and not overcooked. You can eat all the *raw* vegetables you want as long as you include some of all the other basic foods in your diet.

Vegetable Cooking Methods Are Especially Important

How you prepare your vegetables can have much to do with how successful you are on a reducing diet. If you habitually cover raw vegetables with salad dressing, or if you add fat to cooked vegetables, you'll probably gain weight, even if you go on a vegetable diet.

Stan T. included generous amounts of vegetables in his reducing diet. Instead of losing weight, he *gained* weight. "I don't understand it," he said with a puzzled look. "I don't eat sugar. I didn't think vegetables were fattening."

I asked Stan how he prepared his vegetables. "My mother-in-law cooks them," he replied, "and she usually boils them." Further investigation revealed that Stan's mother-in-law seasoned her vegetables very heavily with bacon grease and then boiled them to a mush. The bacon grease added many more calories than the vegetables themselves contained. When Stan eliminated the bacon grease and reduced cooking to a minimum, he began to lose weight.

"I've been losing a couple of pounds a week now for several weeks," Stan reported. "I just didn't realize that cooking methods

would make that much difference. At the rate I'm going now, I'll
get rid of all my excess fat in a couple of months. Incidentally, I like
my vegetables much better when they aren't cooked so much."

How you prepare your foods *does* make a difference. So even
if you balance your diet with the proper food selections, you'll have
to know something about *preparing* your foods, especially your
vegetables, if you want your reducing diet to be effective and
healthful.

How to Steam a Vegetable

The best way to cook a vegetable is to steam it in a colander
that has been placed over a pot of boiling water. Or you may place a
vegetable in a pot that contains just enough water to prevent
scorching and then cover the pot with a tight lid during cooking.
When a vegetable is soft enough to penetrate with a fork, it is
cooked enough.

Overcooking a vegetable—until it is mushy—will not only
destroy nutrients but may also make the vegetable more fattening
by breaking down its cellulose and concentrating its carbohydrate.
Normally, cellulose is indigestible and will pass through the intestinal tract as fiber. But when cellulose is cooked to a mush, it
becomes digestible, thus supplying calories.

Sources of Vitamin C

You can get Vitamin C from such fruits and vegetables as
oranges, grapefruits, cantaloupes, fresh strawberries, broccoli,
brussel sprouts, and peppers. Cabbage, cauliflower, asparagus, collards, garden cress, kale, kohlrabi, mustard greens, potatoes
cooked in their jackets, rutabagas, spinach, tomatoes, and turnip
greens also supply Vitamin C. Obviously, you do not have to depend entirely upon citrus fruit for all of your Vitamin C. Brussels
sprouts and strawberries actually contain *more* Vitamin C than
oranges.

Sources of Vitamin A

The Vitamin A supplied by broccoli, carrots, chard, collards,
cress, kale, pumpkin, sweet potatoes, turnip greens, winter
squash, spinach, apricots, cantaloupe, and other dark green or

deep yellow vegetables can partially replace the Vitamin A you would normally obtain from liver, egg yolk, whole milk, and other fatty animal products. When you reduce your intake of animal fat, you should *increase* your intake of green and yellow vegetables. You should also drink Vitamin A fortified skim milk.

Water-Rich Fruits and Vegetables Are Low in Calories

Except for avocados and olives, fruits and vegetables contain only traces of fat, since they contain a large amount of water. And the leafier the vegetable the more water it contains. A head of lettuce, for example, may be 95 percent water, while potatoes, bananas, winter squash, and more solid fruits and vegetables may be only 70 to 85 percent water. In spite of their high water content, however, leafy vegetables are high in nutrients. The darker, outer leaves contain the greater amount of vitamins and minerals. So be sure to eat the tough outer leaves along with the tender inner leaves.

Although water-rich fruits and vegetables may be rich in nutrients, they are generally low in calories. Remember: The more water a fruit or vegetable contains the lower its calorie content. Tomatoes and oranges, for example, contain fewer calories than potatoes and bananas. *Leafy* vegetables are especially low in calories because of their fiber content as well as because of their water content. Even without the water, the fiber content of fruits and vegetables makes them much less fattening than refined foods.

You don't need to worry about the calorie content of fruits and vegetables in comparing one with another. Both are so much lower in calories than meats and other foods that they can be eaten generously in a balanced diet. Just make sure that you eat your fruits raw and that you cook your vegetables as little as possible.

Eat the Peeling!

Whether you eat your vegetables raw or cooked, don't peel them unless absolutely necessary. The skins of fruits should also be eaten whenever possible. You need the fiber as well as the nutrients supplied by vegetable and fruit skins. Besides, leaving the skin on vegetables during cooking helps prevent loss of nutrients to light, air, and water. When you must cut a vegetable for cooking, cut it into pieces that are just small enough to permit cooking and leave the skin intact.

If you boil a vegetable rather than steam it, use as little water as possible and then use the leftover water as a beverage. Heat will destroy some of the thiamine and Vitamin C, but the water-soluble vitamins and minerals will dissolve into the cooking water to make a nutritious pot liquor. Don't add anything to cooking vegetables except a little salt or plain bouillon. (Some bouillons contain sugar and other ingredients. Be sure to read the label on bouillon cubes before using them as seasoning.) You should not drink pot liquor that has been seasoned with butter, grease, or meat fat.

Adding baking soda or vinegar to preserve the color of a cooked vegetable destroys important vitamins. Adding sugar or fat adds calories. So keep your vegetables plain. Use simple cooking methods. Avoid casseroles and other dishes that contain ingredients other than vegetables.

Cook for One Day at a Time

Cook your vegetables fresh each day so that nutrients won't be lost to overnight storage and reheating. Buy *fresh* vegetables rather than canned, frozen, or precooked vegetables. Remember that even fresh fruits and vegetables lose nutrients when they are stored for several days. Get your produce right from the tree or garden whenever possible. On a low-calorie reducing diet, you'll need all the nutrients you can get from smaller amounts of food.

Overlap Sources of Nutrients

Fresh fruits and vegetables supply such a great variety of nutrients in a balanced diet that they supplement other major sources of nutrients. In addition to supplying Vitamins C and A, for example, fruits supply potassium to balance the sodium supplied by meats. The iron supplied by dried fruit helps replace the iron lost when red meats are eliminated from the diet. Calcium supplied by dark green leafy vegetables helps balance the phosphorus supplied by protein foods. (Spinach, chard, and rhubarb contain oxalic acid which *reduces* absorption of calcium.)

Dark green leafy vegetables also supply iron and some important B vitamins, especially the folic acid you need for the formation of blood cells. The Vitamin B12 you need for healthy blood must come from animal products, however. While both meats and vegetables contribute iron for building and enrichment of blood cells, you must get Vitamin B12 from animal products and folic acid from leafy vegetables to prevent anemia. Obviously, *you cannot depend upon only a few foods for all the essential nutrients as some fad diets suggest.*

When you are on a low-calorie diet that limits food portions, it's especially important to overlap servings of a great variety of foods so that one food complements another. This is one reason why my macro-nutrient diet goes back to the seven basic food groups—to assure the variety you need to protect your health. No one can afford to sacrifice health for quick weight loss.

Remember that while vegetables can supplement meats and dairy products, you should not depend upon vegetables to supply all the iron and calcium you need. If you eat fruits and vegetables, you can eat less meat, but you cannot completely replace animal and dairy products with fruits and vegetables. (See Chapter 5 for a discussion of vegetarianism in a reducing diet.)

THE SPECIAL NUTRIENTS OF WHOLE-GRAIN PRODUCTS

Whole-grain products supply protein, iron, Vitamin E, trace minerals, B vitamins, and some fat as well as complex carbohydrate. They also supply a fiber that's different from the fiber supplied by the cellulose of fruits and vegetables (see Chapter 6). But to get all the benefits of whole grains, you must make sure that the grain products you consume are made from *whole* grains rather than from processed grains. And this requires careful reading of labels.

Wheat: the No. 1 Grain

Wheat is the most popular grain. Unfortunately, most Americans eat *processed* wheat which has had its fiber and most of its nutrients removed. Whole grains (kernels) of wheat are composed of three parts: germ, bran, and endosperm. When wheat is processed, the germ and the bran are removed, leaving only the starchy endosperm. This results in removal of practically all of the wheat's nutrients except carbohydrate and protein. The white flour made from processed wheat is then enriched with iron, thiamine, riboflavin, and niacin, all of which were removed during processing. Many other nutrients lost during processing are not replaced. Chromium, magnesium, zinc, folic acid, Vitamin E, and Vitamin B6, for example, are lost during the processing of wheat kernels. Since wheat is such a big part of our diet, loss of the nutrients supplied by whole wheat could have serious consequences.

There is now some evidence to indicate that chromium deficiency might be a factor in the development of diabetes. Deficiencies in magnesium and Vitamin B6 can contribute to the development of kidney stones and cardiovascular problems. Some nutritionists believe that a low intake of Vitamin E as a result of refining wheat might be partly responsible for the increased incidence of heart disease. Many nutrients that are commonly deficient in our diet could be supplied by whole-wheat products. It would be foolish to substitute processed wheat for whole-grain wheat when you have a choice.

Most nutritionists agree that we should consume a diet that's high in natural carbohydrate. Vegetables and fruits, as you know, should supply the greater part of the carbohydrate in your diet, with whole-grain breads and cereals supplying the balance. Now that we know more about the importance of fiber and the role of trace minerals in the prevention of disease, whole-grain products are being consumed more generously.

Whole Grains Are Less Fattening than Processed Grains

It's the *fiber* in whole grains that makes them less fattening than processed grains. Fiber-rich whole-grain bread, for example, supplies more nutrients and fewer calories than white bread made from refined flour. In addition to providing indigestible bulk, fiber might actually *hinder* absorption of calories. When you are on a reducing diet, you should *always* select whole-grain products rather than the more concentrated refined products. This will increase your intake of fiber and nutrients while *reducing* your intake of calories. Cornmeal, brown barley, oatmeal, brown rice, cracked wheat, whole-wheat bread, shredded wheat, and dark buckwheat and rye flours are examples of whole-grain products. Wheat germ, the most nutritious part of wheat, makes a good cereal—or it can be added to cereals and other foods.

"Quick-cooking" cereals are usually processed and low in fiber. Don't eat them when you have a choice. You should not sacrifice quality for convenience in the kitchen.

Once you become accustomed to the taste of whole-grain products, you'll never again spend your hard-earned money for empty, processed grains. When you buy bread, for example, chances are you'll pass up white bread and look for the coarsest whole-grain bread you can find. You can even find whole-wheat spaghetti and other forms of whole-grain pasta, usually in health food stores.

A Warning About Wheat

While whole-grain wheat is a nutritious food that should be a part of your diet, excessive consumption of wheat might do more harm than good. The phytic acid in wheat and other whole-grain products, for example, tends to reduce absorption of zinc, iron, calcium and a few other minerals—though not to any significant degree, in a *balanced* diet. When you displace other basic foods with wheat, or when you add miller's bran (wheat fiber) to your diet, a problem might develop (see Chapter 6), so keep your diet balanced. Get the fiber you need from fresh fruits and vegetables as well as from whole-grain products.

Much of the phytic acid in whole-wheat bread is destroyed by yeast in the leavening process. It might be a good idea, therefore, to avoid unleavened bread—though cooking grains thoroughly will reduce loss of minerals to phytates.

In addition to containing phytates, whole grains contain little water and are highly concentrated foods. You should never go on an all-grain diet, even temporarily. You should not go on an all-vegetable diet, either. Eating only vegetables will result in deficiencies just as surely as eating only grains or only meat or fruit. Even milk, "the most perfect food," is deficient in iron and Vitamin C. Obviously, it's important to keep your reducing diet balanced with a *variety* of natural foods in order to protect yourself from a nutritional deficiency. This is why my macro-nutrient diet stresses the importance of obtaining energy nutrients from all the basic food groups. Fad diets are usually unbalanced or deficient in essential nutrients.

How to Handle Wheat Allergy

About one person out of every 1,000 is allergic to gluten, a type of protein found in wheat, rye, oats, and barley. The result is celiac disease, or diarrhea, that is characterized by foamy, light-colored stools that contain a considerable amount of fat. Poor absorption of fat-soluble vitamins (A, D, E, and K) and other nutrients leads to the development of anemia, skin disease, soft bones, loose teeth, and other problems.

If you suffer from gluten allergy, you'll have to avoid consuming all grains (and their products) except corn and rice. You might be able to purchase processed gluten-free flour made from the offending grains. Or you can use flour made from corn, rice, soybeans, potatoes, artichokes, and other starchy vegetables in making bread and pasta.

Many processed foods contain "wheat flour," which is actually gluten-rich white flour. Read labels carefully when you purchase packaged products. It's best, of course, to avoid processed foods of any kind. Persons suffering from gluten allergy certainly should not eat processed foods that list wheat flour among their ingredients.

KEEP FATS AND OILS AT A MINIMUM

You should avoid adding fats and oils to your diet. You can get all the fat you need from lean meats and all the oil you need from nuts, seeds, and whole-grain products. You already know that excessive amounts of fats and oils in the diet have been linked to heart disease, cancer, obesity, and other health problems. You must have a certain amount of fat in your diet to supply essential fatty acids and to transport fat-soluble vitamins. And the animal fat in your diet must be balanced with vegetable oil. But if you eat strictly *natural* foods in a balanced diet, using the seven basic food groups as a guide, eliminating all visible fats and oils, you'll get enough fat and you'll automatically balance the fats and oils in your diet. Other than occasional or daily use of a pat of butter on breakfast toast and the use of a tablespoon of vegetable oil as a salad dressing, you do not need additional fat or oil in your diet. The biggest problem with fats and oils is that there is usually *too much* in the diet. So you should make a special effort to eliminate visible fats and oils and then use very little butter, margarine, or cooking oil.

Cooking with Vegetable Oil

When you do need a cooking fat, be sure to use vegetable oil. In addition to being an unsaturated fat, vegetable oil has a higher smoking temperature than animal fat, which means that vegetable oil withstands higher temperatures. Remember, however, that heating a vegetable oil destroys some of its essential fatty acids. Heating an oil until it smokes may break down fatty acids until they become an intestinal irritant.

You should, of course, try to avoid cooking with oil. You can get the essential fatty acids you need by using vegetable oil as a salad dressing. All vegetable oils except coconut oil and olive oil supply essential fatty acids. Safflower and sunflower oils contain the highest percentage of essential linoleic acid.

Vegetable oils also contain Vitamin E, most of which is destroyed during processing. This is unfortunate, since, without the protection of Vitamin E, fatty acids can be oxidized into harmful peroxides in your body. You should never consume rancid oil. Whenever possible, purchase fresh *cold-pressed* oil (available in health food stores).

Wheat germ oil contains more Vitamin E than any other oil.

What About Margarine?

Margarine is simply vegetable oil that has been hardened or saturated by adding hydrogen. The harder the margarine the more saturated it is. Although soft margarines contain a higher percentage of unsaturated fat, you should use margarine sparingly since it contains just as many calories as any fat. Margarine does not contain the cholesterol found in butter and other animal fats, however. This is one reason why most doctors and nutritionists recommend margarine rather than butter. Many persons on a low-fat diet consume fortified margarine for Vitamin A protection. Fortified low-fat milk will supply Vitamin A with fewer calories.

You can keep your intake of fat below the recommended 30 percent of energy intake by using the Table of Nutritive Values in

Chapter 12 to check the fat content of the foods you eat. Try to make sure that you get twice as much fat from vegetable sources as from animal sources. Cutting down on animal fat will automatically reduce your intake of cholesterol and saturated fat. Consuming more unsaturated fat than saturated fat will help keep the fat in your arteries soft and fluid.

Note: Margarine and other forms of hydrogenated vegetable oil contain *trans*-fat, a partially formed fat that might contribute more to the development of cancer, atherosclerosis, and other diseases than naturally saturated fats. So while you should reduce all forms of fat in your diet, it might be best to get the fat you need from such natural foods as nuts, whole milk, eggs, and fresh dairy butter rather than from margarine. Natural fats are also more likely to contain the Vitamin E they need to prevent the oxidation that forms disease-causing lipid oxides.

Remember that hydrogenated peanut butter and shortening, like margarine, contain trans-fat along with saturated fat. Deep-fried foods and *burned* fats (as in charcoal grilling) are rich in toxic lipid oxides. When in doubt, avoid fat. When you have a choice, select a *natural* fat.

Eliminate Visible Meal Fat

You can greatly reduce the calorie content of your diet simply by cutting out visible fats in your meals. A typical steak house meal, for example, consisting of an eight-ounce rib steak, a large baked potato served with butter or sour cream, a tossed salad with French dressing, hot rolls with butter, and coffee with cream and sugar supplies about 1,660 calories. This is far too many calories for one meal. About 1,100 of these calories—67 percent of the total number of calories—come from fat! (Remember that the U.S. Dietary Goals recommend that no more than 30 percent of your calories come from fat.) You can cut these calories in half or more simply by substituting four ounces of broiled fish, poultry, or ground round steak for the eight-ounce rib steak and adding a yellow and a green vegetable (such as squash and green beans). You can do without the butter or sour cream on your baked potato—or you can substitute a pat of margarine. Whole wheat bread could be substituted for rolls and eaten without butter. A little lemon juice with vinegar can be used as a salad dressing. You can drink coffee without sugar and cream—or, better yet, you can drink water, skim milk, unsweetened tea, or tomato juice. You may then have a piece of fresh fruit for dessert.

In addition to lowering calories and increasing fiber, such dietary changes as those I have just outlined will greatly decrease your intake of saturated fat and cholesterol and provide a better balance between saturated fat and unsaturated fat. Best of all, you'll be able to eat a greater amount of food.

Simply making an effort to eliminate visible fats and oils in your diet and selecting low-fat *natural* foods will cut your calorie intake enough to assure weight loss in most cases. But you must cook without fat or oil and avoid sugar and white flour products if you're really serious about dieting. And you must balance your diet with fruits, vegetables, grains, and dairy products—with emphasis on vegetables.

Once you get your weight down, you can have a little sugar occasionally—if you still have a taste for it.

SUMMARY

1. *All of the nutrients you need for good health must be obtained from foods rather than from supplements.*
2. *How you prepare your foods can be just as important as selection of foods in getting adequate nutrients on a low-calorie diet.*
3. *Vitamin A and D fortified low-fat milk and its products supply all the nutrients of whole milk with fewer calories.*
4. *Persons who suffer from lactose intolerance should switch to fermented skim milk products.*
5. *Iron-rich soybeans can be substituted for red meats in a diet that is balanced with other basic foods.*
6. *It's essential that you include such animal products as skim milk, cottage cheese, poultry, eggs, or fish in your diet for Vitamin B_{12} and other essential B vitamins.*
7. *Both fruits and vegetables supply carbohydrate with Vitamin C and Vitamin A, but you should depend more upon fruits for Vitamin C and more upon vegetables for Vitamin A.*
8. *Fruits should always be eaten raw. Vegetables that cannot be eaten raw should be cooked with as little heat, water, and time as possible.*
9. *Whole-grain products are good sources of protein and fiber as well as Vitamin E, complex carbohydrate, minerals, and other essential nutrients.*
10. *You can get all the fat and oil you need from a balanced diet of low-fat natural foods without adding fat or oil to your foods.*

5

Special Macro-Nutrient
Food Sources of Healthful,
Low-Fat Protein

Have you seen some of those reducing diets that recommend exotic dishes composed of strange, hard-to-find foods? I never could understand why anyone would devise a diet that calls for consumption of anything other than simple, basic foods. To succeed on any diet, you must eat foods that are readily available and easy to prepare. You must be able to select foods that you enjoy eating. If you pick the foods you like best from each of the seven basic food groups and then prepare them in the simplest way possible, food selection and preparation won't be a problem. You can't go wrong with such foods as broiled fish, steamed vegetables, green salads, skim milk, fresh fruits, and whole-grain bread and cereals.

As you know from reading Chapter 4, there are some unusual foods that may occasionally be substituted for some of the more common basic foods. Soybeans, for example, are sometimes substituted for red meats. Persons lacking a certain digestive enzyme must substitute fermented milk products for fresh milk. Vegetarians must combine grains and legumes and other dishes to replace meat protein. Although all fish are lower in fat than meats, some fish contain more oil than others, thus providing you with a choice.

In this chapter, I'll tell you how to cook soybeans, how to combine grains and beans for a complete protein, how to make your own whole-grain bread, how to cultivate low-fat yogurt, how to grow vitamin-rich sprouts, and how to prepare other unusual foods that contribute something special in a reducing diet. I'll also tell you how to select and combine foods for vegetarian-type meals. What you learn in this chapter will provide the variety you need to make your diet more interesting. Furthermore, such kitchen projects as making bread and yogurt and growing sprouts will prove to be an exciting challenge.

How Denise Lost 44 Pounds on a Special Variation of Macro-Nutrient Dieting

Denise F. was 44 pounds overweight and knew very little about how to eat properly. "I'm going to quit eating meat," she announced. "I want to become a vegetarian!"

There is, of course, more to becoming a vegetarian than just eliminating meat from the diet, especially on a low-calorie reducing diet. When I finished lecturing Denise on the importance of protein in the diet and the dangers of strict vegetarianism, she recanted. "Well, what I'd really like to do is become a lacto-ovo-vegetarian," she said, revealing a knowledge of nutrition.

Even though Denise eliminated red meats from her diet, she was able to get all the protein, iron, and other nutrients she needed from other foods in a balanced diet. She got rid of 44 pounds in 14 weeks without jeopardizing her health.

"I've never been on such an interesting and versatile diet," Denise said enthusiastically. "I'm preparing all my own foods. I'm even baking my own bread! I've replaced meat with a small amount of fish, but I'm fascinated by the art of obtaining a complete protein from a combination of grains and vegetables. What I like most about my macro-nutrient diet, however, is that it's flexible enough to allow for intelligent adjustments in meeting the needs of the individual—meat eater, vegetarian, or whatever."

After you read this chapter, you'll have the knowledge and the skill you need to make special adjustments in your diet. You'll amaze and entertain your family and your friends by preparing unusual, highly nutritious "diet dishes."

SUBSTITUTING SOYBEANS FOR MEAT

Dry soybeans contain eleven times more fat than other types of beans, but they contain less fat and fewer calories than meat. They also contain 1½ times more protein than other beans—and their protein is nearly equal to that of meat. Unlike meat fat, however, soybean fat is unsaturated. This is one reason why soybean products are often substituted for meat.

Green soybeans supply some of the Vitamin A that's missing in a low-fat diet, but they lose most of this vitamin when they are dried. Soybeans and other legumes do supply iron, however, and they help supply the iron you lose when you remove red meat from your diet. One cup of cooked legumes, for example, supplies about 31 percent of the protein and 42 percent of the iron needed daily by adults.

People used to believe that all beans were fattening. We now know that this is not true. In addition to supplying important fiber and complex carbohydrate, beans, especially soybeans, are a low-calorie source of high-quality protein. Remember, however, that the protein supplied by beans must be complemented with protein supplied by milk, grains, and other foods in a balanced diet.

Warning: Although most vegetables may be eaten raw, soybeans and other beans should always be *cooked*. Raw beans contain toxins that might interfere with digestion; they also contain phytates that hinder absorption of zinc and other minerals.

How to Cook Fresh Soybeans

Fresh, green soybeans make a tasty, succulent vegetable, but they are available only in some areas of the country in late summer or fall. *Vegetable* soybeans are used for cooking. They are larger and have a milder flavor than the *field* soybeans used for oil and flour. Vegetable soybeans may be picked for cooking when their pods are bright green. The pods, however, are not edible.

It's much easier to shell fresh soybeans if you'll first let them soak in boiling water for five minutes. Then, after pouring off the water and letting the beans cool, you can break open the pods and squeeze out the beans.

To cook shelled green soybeans, add two cups of beans to one cup of boiling water. Add one-half teaspoon of salt for seasoning if desired. Bring the water to a boil, cover the pot, and cook gently for 10 to 20 minutes until the beans are tender.

Cooked, fresh soybeans resemble green peas or lima beans in color and flavor but have a firmer texture.

If green soybeans are not available fresh, you can purchase them canned and precooked. Canned soybeans are commonly substituted for lima beans in casseroles and other dishes.

Cooking Dry Soybeans

Dry soybeans require much more soaking and cooking than the fresh variety. Be sure to *wash* the beans before soaking—and remember that one cup of dry soybeans will yield about 2½ cups of cooked beans.

The quickest way to soak soybeans is to boil them for two minutes and then let them stand for one hour after removing them from the stove. It will be necessary to use four cups of water for each cup of dry beans to allow for expansion of the beans during soaking and cooking. After the beans have soaked, add one teaspoon of salt for each cup of beans. Then cover the pot and simmer for two to three hours until the beans are tender. You may add as much water as necessary to keep the beans submerged while cooking.

Drain the beans you put on your plate—and discard the cooking water. You should *not* drink the water used to cook soybeans.

Cooked dry soybeans taste very much like boiled peanuts. And they are firm and chewy. They provide a nutritious taste treat that will enhance anyone's diet.

How to Grow Vitamin-Rich Soy Sprouts

When any seed, grain, or legume is sprouted, its nutrient values are greatly increased. Soybeans are no exception. When dry soybeans are sprouted, the sprouts actually *manufacture* vitamins! Sprouted soybeans also contain fewer calories, since they contain less fat and carbohydrate. A cupful of sprouted beans, for example, supplies only 48 calories but as much protein as an egg which supplies 80 calories. Great fuel for your reducing power pedal!

Grain sprouts are usually eaten raw in salads and on sandwiches. But soybean sprouts should be cooked or steamed a little to increase their digestibility and to destroy harmful enzymes. The process of sprouting soybeans will neutralize most of their toxins and phytates. To be on the safe side, however, you should *cook* sprouted beans before eating them.

When soybeans sprout, they increase in volume about six times. One-third cup of dry beans, for example, will yield about two cups of sprouts.

Basically, all you have to do to sprout beans is place them in a container that has good drainage so that you can rinse them with cool water four or five times a day. A clean clay flower pot lined with cheesecloth (to cover the hole in the bottom of the pot), or a milk carton with small holes punched in its sides and bottom, will do fine. Just make sure that the container is large enough to accommodate the sprouting beans.

First soak the beans overnight in water. Use three times as much water as beans in order to provide adequate water for absorption. Rinse the beans before placing them in a pre-prepared sprouting container. Then place the container in a dark, cool place (about 65 degrees Fahrenheit) or cover it with a damp towel. Rinse the beans several times a day by running water through the container. This will wash away mold and encourage sprouting. It's important to make sure that the water drains freely and that air can circulate through the container. (The same sprouting technique can be used to sprout any edible seed or grain, such as alfalfa or wheat.)

How to Cook Bean Sprouts

After three or four days, when the sprouts are two or three inches long, the sprouted beans may be rinsed, cooked, and eaten. Two cups of raw sprouts will yield one cup of cooked sprouts. The sprouted beans should be cooked just enough to destroy the enzymes in the bean but not so much that you destroy the Vitamin C in the sprout.

To parboil (partly cook) sprouted soybeans, drop them into boiling water, using one-half cup of water and one-quarter teaspoon of salt for each cup of sprouts. Boil gently for 10 minutes or so until the sprouts are tender but still crisp. Soybean sprouts, drained and lightly seasoned with lemon juice, make a good protein-rich vegetable dish, or they can be added to salads.

Replacing Cow's Milk with Soy Milk

In Chapter 4, I mentioned that persons allergic to cow's milk might want to substitute soy milk to assure an adequate intake of calcium and protein. Soy milk can replace cow's milk in most recipes and can be used as a beverage. You can purchase soy milk (usually in dry form) that has been fortified with Vitamin B_{12} and other nutrients to approximate the composition of cow's milk. Vegetarians who do not consume animal products may substitute fortified soy milk for cow's milk to guard against a Vitamin B_{12} deficiency.

If you want to know more about how to cook with soybeans or how to make your own soy milk, write the Superintendent of Documents, U.S. Government Printing Office, Washington, D.C. 20402 and ask for the booklet *Soybeans,* Home and Garden Bulletin No. 208.

FISH SUPPLIES FEWER CALORIES THAN MEAT

On a low-fat macro-nutrient diet, you should eat fresh fish often, since it is an excellent source of low-fat protein. And the fat it does contain is *unsaturated.* Fish also supplies Vitamin B_{12}, iron, Vitamin D, and varying amounts of Vitamin A, all of which tend to be in short supply in a diet that excludes fat-rich meat. Salt water fish are a good source of iodine and, like all fish, are low in sodium. This makes ocean fish especially useful when iodized salt must be eliminated in a low-sodium (low-salt) diet.

Although some fish contain more oil than others, *all fish and shellfish are low in fat and contain fewer calories than beef or pork.* Even the fattest fish rarely contain more than 10 percent fat, with many fish averaging less than one percent fat. Pork may contain up to 49 percent fat and beef up to 43 percent fat. If you cook without grease or oil, you can reduce your calorie intake by substituting any kind of fish or shellfish for meat.

Shellfish tend to be high in cholesterol, but they are also rich in minerals. Oysters, for example, are extremely rich in iron, zinc, and copper. Shellfish also supply fewer calories than other forms of fish. Because of their cholesterol content, however, shellfish must be eaten sparingly by persons suffering from high blood cholesterol.

You may eat fish every day if you like. If you do, you might want to select a low-fat variety. Flounder, haddock, Atlantic cod, tuna, and red snapper, for example, are low in fat, while Atlantic herring and Atlantic mackerel contain a little more fat.

The U.S. Department of Agriculture rates popular fish and shellfish according to grams of fat (percentage of fat) per 100 grams of fish. (See Table 5-1.)

100 Grams of Fish	Grams of Fat
Eel, American	18.3
Herring, Atlantic	16.4
Mackerel, Atlantic	9.8
Tuna, albacore (canned, light)	6.8
Tuna, albacore (white meat)	8.0
Salmon, sockeye	8.9
Salmon, Atlantic	5.8
Carp	6.2
Rainbow trout (U.S.)	4.5
Striped bass	2.1
Ocean perch	2.5
Red snapper	1.2
Tuna, skipjack (canned, light)	.8
Halibut, Atlantic	1.1
Cod, Atlantic	.7
Haddock	.7

100 Grams of Shellfish	Grams of Fat
Eastern oyster	2.1
Pacific oyster	2.3
Ark shell clam	1.5
Blue crab	1.6
Alaska king crab	1.6
Shrimp	1.2
Scallop	.9

Table 5-1

You can further reduce the fat content of fish by removing the skin, which is higher in fat than the flesh. When you buy canned fish such as tuna, select a variety packed in water if it is available. Canned fish that includes the bones of the fish, as in salmon or sardines, will provide calcium as a nutritional bonus.

HOW TO MAKE YOUR OWN LOW-FAT YOGURT

Whether you eat yogurt because you can't digest milk sugar or simply because you enjoy the taste of fermented milk, you should make your own yogurt if you want to make sure that it is alive and fresh and low in calories. The live bacteria in yogurt will make a healthful contribution to your intestinal tract. The lactic acid produced by these bacteria will aid digestion and improve absorption of nutrients.

Unfortunately, yogurt containing live bacteria does not have a long shelf life. The older a live yogurt the stronger and more watery it becomes because of continued bacterial activity. For this reason, some commercial manufacturers of yogurt kill the bacteria with heat or paralyze them with additives and preservatives. Otherwise, yogurt could not be so easily stored and shipped around the nation.

You can get all the benefits of live yogurt if you make your own at home using nothing but skim milk and a bacterial culture. Fresh yogurt goes great with fresh fruit, sliced vegetables, seeds, nuts, cereals, or any other healthful food of your choice. Or you may simply eat yogurt by itself. Yogurt made from skim milk provides all the nutrients of skim milk—with a few special benefits.

Unique Properties of Yogurt

When a bacterial culture is added to milk, some of the Vitamin B_{12} in the milk is used by the bacteria in converting lactose (milk sugar) to lactic acid. But the benefits of yogurt far outweigh this slight loss. The protein in yogurt, for example, is more digestible than the protein in milk. The bacteria in live yogurt displace harmful bacteria in the intestinal tract. Lactobacillus (yogurt bacteria) also produces an acid that inhibits the growth of disease-producing bacteria.

It's well known that taking oral antibiotics kills healthful intestinal bacteria along with infecting bacteria. When your doctor prescribes antibiotics to kill an infection, you can help restore intestinal bacteria by eating fresh, live yogurt. If you can make your own yogurt at home, so much the better.

Technique for Making Yogurt

For yogurt culture to grow successfully, the milk containing the culture must be kept warm for several hours—until the milk congeals or thickens. If you don't have a commercial yogurt maker, you'll have to devise other ways to keep the milk heated to a temperature of about 110 degrees Fahrenheit. If the temperature goes below 90 degrees or above 120 degrees, the bacteria won't multiply. You can heat cultured milk by placing it on a rack above the eye of a stove, in a box containing an electric light bulb, on top of an electric blanket, or in some other warm place. Obviously, you can more effectively control the temperature of the fermenting milk by using a commercial yogurt maker.

Before you add yogurt bacteria to milk, it would be a good idea to first heat the milk to the boiling point (at least to 180 degrees) to kill all the competing bacteria. Cool the milk down to 110 degrees Fahrenheit before adding the bacterial culture. If you prefer, you may use a couple of tablespoons of fresh yogurt as a starter.

You can make yogurt in one big batch in a covered pot or you can make it in several small covered containers. It might be easier, however, to maintain a uniformly desirable temperature in the smaller containers. When the yogurt has congealed and the flavor is just right, you can prevent further fermentation by placing the yogurt in a refrigerator. Remember that the longer milk ferments the stronger the flavor. If you like your yogurt firm and sweet, add powdered non-fat milk along with the bacterial culture and stop the fermentation as soon as the milk congeals.

Growing and eating yogurt is a fascinating, healthful practice that will provide a positive stimulus in your weight-reducing program. Tending to your yogurt will provide the psychological lift you'd get from regular visits to a doctor, a hypnotist, a spa, or a weight club. Involvement in any activity that requires you to help yourself in reaching your weight goal will help assure success.

WHOLE-GRAIN HOMEMADE BREAD IS BEST!

When you order whole-wheat bread in restaurants, they usually bring you caramel-colored "wheat bread" made from white flour. One reason for this is that such bread has a longer shelf life and doesn't spoil easily—and it's cheaper. Real whole-wheat bread that does not contain additives and preservatives must be kept refrigerated to retard molding.

If you want some really good bread, you should make your own. In addition to being healthful, homemade whole-grain bread is tasty and low in calories. You can add bran, raisins, soy flour, bone meal, nuts, powdered skim milk, or anything you like to make the bread super nutritious. Adding two tablespoons of powdered skim milk to one cup of whole-wheat flour, for example, will greatly increase the protein quality of the bread. A little soy flour added to wheat flour will make the bread moist and chewy and enrich it with calcium and protein. You can add bran for additional fiber.

The natural carbohydrate of protein-rich whole-wheat bread is a great protein-sparing fuel for your body's fat-burner throttle.

Everyone should experience the taste of fiber-rich homemade bread. I have included my recipe for whole-wheat bread in many of my books on nutrition. Almost without exception, persons who start making their own bread never again buy a loaf of white bread.

Whole-Grain Bread Is Not Fattening!

Whole-grain bread is not nearly as fattening as most people think. In fact, when bread is coarse and rich in fiber, it is one of the least fattening and the most satisfying of all the natural foods. Since you should have four or more servings of a whole-grain product each day to balance your diet, you can have at least one slice of whole-wheat bread with each meal in addition to your morning cereal. When you include homemade whole-grain bread in your diet, chances are you'll eat less of other foods because of the satiety value of bread.

Actually, it's all right to eat extra slices of whole-grain bread as long as your total calorie intake does not exceed the number you need to reach your weight goal or to maintain your ideal weight. Professor Olaf Mickelsen of Michigan State University, quoted in *Dietary Goals for the United States*, reported that bread in large amounts is an ideal food in a weight-reducing program. "Recent work in our laboratory indicates that slightly overweight young men lost weight in a painless and practically effortless manner when they included 12 slices of bread per day in their program,"

Dr. Mickelsen observed. "That bread was eaten with their meals. As a result, they became satisfied before they consumed their usual quota of calories. The subjects were admonished to restrict those foods that were concentrated sources of energy; otherwise, they were free to eat as much as they desired. In eight weeks, the average weight loss for each subject was 12.7 pounds."

It's important to make sure that the bread you eat is *whole-grain* in order to be assured of an adequate intake of vitamins, minerals, and fiber. The more fiber your bread contains, the fewer calories it supplies.

You'll learn more in the next chapter about how to increase your intake of fiber in natural foods for faster weight loss. In the meantime, you can enrich homemade whole-wheat bread with fiber by adding a little miller's bran.

My Favorite Homemade Whole-Wheat Bread Recipe

Whole-grain wheat flour is rich in fiber, but it's always a good idea to add a little extra fiber by mixing a few tablespoons of miller's bran into the bread dough. You can reduce the calorie value of your bread by substituting one-half cup of miller's bran for one-half cup of flour in each recipe.

Here's my favorite bread recipe:

Mix 3 cups of warm water with ½ cup of honey and 2 packages of baker's yeast. Allow this mixture to stand for 5 minutes or longer and then add 5 cups of unsifted stone-ground whole-wheat flour.

Beat this mixture by hand 100 times or more.

Add 2 or 3 additional cups of whole-wheat flour (or enough to make the dough stiff) and 1 scant tablespoon of salt.

Knead the dough until it is smooth and elastic, adding enough flour to prevent sticking.

Place the dough in an oiled bowl in a warm place and let the dough rise until it doubles in bulk.

Knead the dough back to its original size and place it in two 1½-pound loaf pans that have been greased with margarine.

Let the dough rise until it reaches the top of the pan before placing it in the oven.

Bake in a preheated oven at 350 degrees Fahrenheit for about 60 minutes or until the bread is well-browned.

VEGETARIANISM IN A REDUCING DIET

A vegetarian diet is essentially a high-carbohydrate diet consisting of fruits, vegetables, seeds, nuts, and grains. Such a diet has proved to be non-fattening. You never see a fat vegetarian.

Actually, there are several varieties of vegetarianism. A true vegetarian who eats only foods of plant origin is called a *vegan*. A *lacto-vegetarian* includes milk and its products. An *ovo-vegetarian* includes eggs. An *ovo-lacto-vegetarian* includes both eggs and milk. Some vegetarians eat fish. Many people who eliminate red meats from their diet call themselves vegetarians. *The one thing that all vegetarians have in common is that they do not eat the flesh of warmblooded creatures.*

Because of the high saturated fat and cholesterol content of red meats, most of us would do well to eat less red meat. If you don't eat poultry, you should at least eat fish. It's absolutely essential that the average person include eggs or milk products—or both—in a vegetarian diet to assure an adequate intake of Vitamin B_{12}. You already know from reading earlier chapters of this book that you must make a special effort to increase your intake of iron and fat-soluble vitamins when you eliminate red meat and animal fat from your diet. When you eliminate *all* animal products from your diet, including fish, dairy products, and eggs, you must supplement your diet with Vitamin B_{12} and possibly calcium. You must also learn how to combine grains and legumes (such as rice and beans) and other vegetables to form a complete protein that can be used by your body to build tissue. And you must seek out seeds and plant foods that are rich in calcium.

Balancing a Vegetarian Reducing Diet

A true vegetarian who wants to stay healthy must select and combine foods carefully, and this requires considerable study. A vegetarian must also eat large quantities of a great variety of vegetables and grains each day to supply adequate protein—and this may require a great deal of eating between meals. One popular vegetarian reducing diet requires you to eat four pounds of food a day in eight meals to supply only 700 calories and 35 grams of protein—both too low for the best of health.

Most of us would prefer to include fish, eggs, and milk products for nutritional insurance and to provide the protein, iron, and calcium we need without eating so much. This is one reason why I balance my macro-nutrient diet with animal products. If you want to eat between meals to satisfy your urge to nibble on something, you can't go wrong with raw vegetables. You won't be able to eat enough of them to hurt your diet (see Chapter 7). During regular meals, however, it would be best to include fish, eggs, poultry, or skim milk products with other basic foods. Vegetarians who are not intolerant of the lactose in milk can use milk to complete the protein in their diet as well as to provide Vitamin B12.

A Vegetarian Food Plan

Here is a basic four food group plan developed at the University of Florida for vegetarians:

2 servings of milk or milk products (or soy milk fortified with Vitamin B12)

2 servings of protein-rich foods (include 2 cups of legumes daily to help meet iron requirements for women; count 4 tablespoons of peanut butter as one serving)

4 servings of whole-grain foods

4 servings of fruits and vegetables (include 1 cup of dark greens to help meet iron requirements for women)

Since vegetables and grains contain an incomplete protein, you must combine grains (such as corn, rice, and wheat) and legumes (peas and beans) *in each meal* to provide a complete protein. Combining seeds and nuts with legumes also helps form a complete protein. Eating grains or seeds in the morning and legumes in the evening won't meet your needs. Plant proteins must be combined *in the same meal* if they are to be used by your body to form a complete protein. One solution to the problem of combining plant proteins would be to include a small amount of milk, fish, or cottage cheese in each meal to contribute the amino acids your body needs to form a complete protein from the incomplete protein supplied by plant foods. But that would not be a true vegetarian meal.

If you want to eat the vegetarian way for a couple of days, include a dish that combines brown rice with your favorite bean. Combining three-fourths cup of beans with two cups of rice will supply about the same amount of protein as a 9½-ounce steak at about one fourth the price.

Soybeans, as you know, provide a complete protein. Commercial soy products that taste like meat and supply all the nutrients of meat can be purchased in most grocery stores.

Peanut butter on whole-grain bread will provide a complete protein. So will corn bread and peas. You can make corn bread into a complete protein by mixing sesame seeds with corn meal.

Planning True Vegetarian Meals

True vegetarians can meet their protein requirement in each meal by including a serving of legumes (beans) and grains at noon and evening meals and a serving of whole-grain cereal with seeds and nuts at breakfast. Your favorite seed or nut butter on whole-grain bread will also supply a complete protein. Tahini, for example, which is made by grinding toasted sesame seeds into a mush, can be spread on bread or mixed into a soy milk shake for extra protein and calcium. The protein in sesame seeds combines especially well with the protein provided by soybeans.

Servings of fruits can complete the morning meal, while servings of vegetables and whole-grain bread can complete noon and evening meals. If you include a little Vitamin B_{12}-enriched soy milk at breakfast and at one other meal, you can assure an adequate intake of protein and Vitamin B_{12} without consuming animal products.

Wheat germ and brewer's yeast supply complete protein as well as some Vitamin B_{12}. Both of these products make ideal supplements in a vegetarian meal. Wheat germ can be eaten as a cereal or it can be added to cereals. Yeast can be taken in tablet form or mixed into vegetable juice with a blender. I prefer to add yeast powder to whole-grain cereal and to peanut butter. I also use yeast power in energy drinks.

Note: Although the vegetarian way of eating is an effective way to reduce excess body fat, I do not recommend that the average person stay on a true vegetarian diet for more than a few days at a time.

Gavin MacLeod of TV's "Love Boat" reduced his body weight from 265 pounds to 184 pounds on a vegetarian diet. But he was careful to include eggs, fish, and other animal products to assure an adequate intake of protein and Vitamin B$_{12}$. I'd suggest that you do the same.

COMPLETE MEAL IN A SALAD

If you don't like to cook and you'd like to occasionally substitute a raw salad for a cooked meal, you can do so if you prepare a salad that contains all the ingredients of a balanced meal. This won't be hard to do if you use the basic four food groups as a guide. If you're not a true vegetarian, you can meet your protein requirement simply by mixing in a little cottage cheese, broiled fish, or diced poultry.

For most of us, the main ingredients of any salad are lettuce and tomatoes. And that's fine. But don't fill your bowl too full with lettuce. Leave room for a variety of other vegetables. You can get more Vitamin A, calcium, and iron from the darker-leaved vegetables, such as kale, parsley, spinach, and watercress. Always select a darker variety of lettuce rather than iceberg and other light lettuces. Use the darker outer leaves whenever possible. The dark green flower buds of broccoli as well as the flowerets of cauliflower can be eaten raw in salads.

Remember that while leafy vegetables are rich in vitamins and minerals, they contain more water and fiber than anything else. So you'll have to include a *variety* of vegetables to get sufficient carbohydrate. Carrots, celery, sweet potatoes, sprouts, onions, radishes, and other favorite vegetables can be included in a raw salad. But don't forget: no raw beans! If you include soybean sprouts, cook or steam them a little before eating them.

How to Enrich Your Salads

Sunflower seeds can be added to salads for additional protein, carbohydrate, oil, and Vitamin D as well as for a crunchy taste treat. You can even throw in a little wheat germ for B vitamins and Vitamin E. Most vegetables supply Vitamin C as well as Vitamin A, but you can include strawberries, orange slices, lemon juice, or pineapple for a sweet source of Vitamin C. Diced apples and raisins are good sweeteners. A small amount of broiled fish, baked chicken, boiled egg, or uncreamed cottage cheese mixed into your salad will provide a complete protein. I prefer cottage cheese, since it supplies calcium as well as protein. I then add a boiled egg for nutritional insurance.

All salads should be prepared fresh and eaten immediately if possible. Cutting vegetables and letting them stand results in loss of nutrients. If you have leftover salad, cover it and keep it in the refrigerator until your next meal.

Actress Michele Lee of the "Knots Landing" TV series often has only salad for dinner. "I *love* salads," she says enthusiastically. "I put *everything* in my salads—sunflower seeds or nuts, crepes, raisins, cheese, tomatoes, fresh cauliflower or broccoli, and so on."

With a little imagination, you can make a complete, nutritious meal in salad form, and you can select the foods you like best. When you don't have a wide variety of foods to choose from, just try to include a dark green leafy vegetable, a little cottage cheese or a boiled egg, and a few raw sunflower seeds to a bowl of lettuce and tomatoes. Lemon juice can be used as a dressing. Skim milk would be an ideal beverage. You may then have a piece of fresh fruit for dessert—or you may select dried fruit for additional iron.

One-half cup of uncreamed cottage cheese supplies about 17 grams of protein and 90 milligrams of calcium. One cup of nonfat milk supplies nine grams of protein and 296 milligrams of calcium. This is enough protein and calcium for one meal. Sunflower seeds are about 30 percent protein and are rich in iron, Vitamin D, and essential fatty acids.

A salad consisting of four lettuce leaves (40 calories), one tomato (40 calories), one-half cup of uncreamed cottage cheese (85 calories), and three tablespoons of sunflower seeds (63 calories), with one cup of skim milk as a beverage (90 calories) and an apple as a dessert (70 calories), will supply less than 400 calories.

Although salads can be enriched with calcium and protein, you should not try to get by on salads alone. You also need some cooked foods. Have a salad every day, but only occasionally substitute a salad for a complete meal.

HEALTH DRINKS SUBSTITUTED FOR MEALS

High-protein energy drinks are commonly used as meal substitutes on a reducing diet. Such drinks are usually too unbalanced, however, to depend upon for your daily quota of nutrients, even when supplemented with vitamins and minerals. Remember that about 58 *percent of your energy intake should come from natural carbohydrate for the best of health* (with at least 60 grams of protein daily to maintain lean body tissue).

Your body *must* have adequate carbohydrate to burn for energy if it is to function efficiently, and this carbohydrate must supply fiber as well as nutrients. For this reason, *you should never substitute a protein drink for more than one meal a day.* The other two meals should supply the fiber and everything else your body needs in a balanced diet.

You'll remember that in Chapter 1 I said that you need at least 100 grams of *complex* carbohydrate daily for good health. If you have a high-protein drink for breakfast, you should be sure to include fruits, vegetables, and whole grains in your noon and evening meals. The total number of calories you take in during the day will determine the extent of your weight loss. So you'll still have to watch your calories, even if you substitute a low-calorie protein drink for one meal.

Basic Formula for an Energy Drink

Basically, a high-protein energy drink usually consists of nothing more than skim milk, protein powder, and brewer's yeast. Milk supplies some carbohydrate. *Fresh fruit or unsweetened fruit juice concentrate may be added for additional carbohydrate* as well as for Vitamin C. Mix all this with several ice cubes in a blender and you have a cold, creamy, low-calorie milk shake.

If you prefer, you may use powdered skim milk or soy powder instead of protein powder. Skim milk powder can be purchased in any grocery store. You can add eight grams of protein and 12 grams of carbohydrate to an eight-ounce glass of skim milk simply by stirring in five level tablespoons of nonfat dry milk. This will add up to about 17 grams of protein and 24 grams of carbohydrate in the milk itself. Persons who cannot digest milk sugar can use soy milk mixed with soy powder or a commercial high-protein powder that does not contain milk powder.

The brewer's yeast in an energy drink supplies an antifatigue factor as well as B vitamins that help the body produce energy. Until you become accustomed to the taste of yeast, you can use only a small amount of yeast powder to begin with. You may then gradually increase the amount of yeast you use according to your taste.

Here's a simple recipe for mixing a supply of energy drinks:

> *1 quart skim milk*
> *½ cup brewer's yeast powder*
> *½ cup skim milk powder*
> *1 small can frozen fruit juice concentrate*

Mix all these ingredients in a blender and store them in a refrigerator. Each time you pour a glass of the mixture, remix the serving with ice cubes in a blender.

Doctor Homola's Meal-Substitute Energy Drink

Here's the formula I follow in making my own low-calorie energy drink:

> *1 cup (8 ounces) of skim milk (9 grams of protein, 12 grams of carbohydrate, and 90 calories)*
> *1 heaping tablespoon of protein powder (15 grams of protein and 60 calories)*
> *2 level teaspoons of brewer's yeast powder (3 grams of protein, 3 grams of carbohydrate, and 25 calories)*
> *1 banana (1 gram of protein, 26 grams of carbohydrate, and 100 calories)*
> *8 to 10 ice cubes*
> *Vanilla flavoring if desired*

All of these ingredients mixed in a blender will make a little more than two cups for a total of 28 grams of protein, 41 grams of carbohydrate, and 275 calories. The more ice you add, the thicker the drink and the fewer calories per ounce. This drink provides a filling meal for so few calories. You may not be able to drink all the mixture at one meal. So adjust your recipe accordingly.

You may, of course, use any fruit you like in an energy drink. Most fruits supply fewer calories than a banana. An apple, for example, supplies about 70 calories, an orange about 65 calories, a cup of diced pineapple about 75 calories, a peach about 35 calories, and a cup of fresh strawberries about 55 calories. It really doesn't matter what kind of fruit you use. The calories and carbohydrate supplied by any fresh fruit won't be excessive.

How Jean Used Energy Drinks to Lose 33 Pounds

Jean A. wanted to lose as much weight as she could as rapidly as possible. She took the 1,200 calorie three-meal diet outlined in Chapter 3 and substituted a high-protein energy drink for *one meal* a day. Sometimes she substituted the drink for breakfast, other times for lunch or dinner, depending upon how her job as a TV reporter affected scheduled meals. She also took a multiple vitamin and mineral supplement.

Jean's meal plan allowed only about 900 calories a day. Since her ideal weight was about 130 pounds, she would normally require about 2,000 calories to maintain that weight. With a deficit of 1,100 calories a day, Jean expected to lose only a little more than two pounds a week. Instead, she lost 10 pounds in two weeks! Since some of Jean's weight loss might have been body water, I advised her to go back to a three-meal 1,200 calorie diet. Her weight loss slowed to two or three pounds a week. In 12 weeks, she had permanently reduced from a chubby 162 pounds to a full, firm 129 pounds.

If you use energy drinks as a meal substitute, try to eat at least two conventional meals a day. No kind of meal substitute should ever replace more than. two meals a day—and only then for no longer than two weeks at a time. If you take in only 600 calories or less a day with meal substitutes, you'll lose weight fast, but it won't all be fat. Worst of all, you might damage your health, even if you take supplements. So don't take any chances. Stick to the diet plan outlined earlier in this book and use energy drinks only occasionally as a meal substitute.

Enriching Energy Drinks with Vitamins

During the winter months when you may need additional Vitamin C to combat colds, it might be a good idea to use strawberries or oranges in your energy drinks. One cup of strawberries supplies 88 milligrams of Vitamin C, more than any other fruit. An orange supplies 66 milligrams of Vitamin C, a banana 12 milligrams of Vitamin C, and an apple only three milligrams of Vitamin C. Whenever possible, *it's best to use whole fruit rather than juice in order to boost your intake of fiber* along with Vitamin C and carbohydrate.

"I get my vitamins in health drinks, which I love," says actor Peter Lawford, who substitutes a health drink for one meal each day. "Sometimes I make my drink with orange juice and milk. I add protein powder, a couple of eggs, a banana, or sometimes a few strawberries for a different taste. To me, a health drink is a great way to get going in the morning. Sometimes I have the drink for lunch—whenever I feel like it. Sometimes I add brewer's yeast. I use a soy protein powder that has everything in it—all the vitamins and minerals."

You can make your own health drink to suit your needs and your taste, and you may occasionally use it as a meal substitute to speed weight loss. Remember, however, that it's not a good idea to take in fewer than 1,200 calories a day, even on a reducing diet. When health drinks are substituted for more than one meal a day, calorie intake may fall below 1,000 calories a day. This is one reason why such drinks result in faster weight loss and why they must be accompanied by vitamin and mineral supplements.

Pure protein drinks, such as liquid protein, should be avoided altogether. When there is too much protein and not enough carbohydrate, excessive loss of body water drains nutrients from the body, resulting in dangerous deficiencies.

SUMMARY

1. *Whenever possible, a reducing diet should consist of favorite foods selected from all the basic food groups.*
2. *Except in the case of true vegetarianism, an animal product such as skim milk, cottage cheese, fish, or eggs should supply most of the protein your body needs.*
3. *In a vegetarian diet, cooked soybeans can be substituted for meat. Fortified soy milk can replace cow's milk.*
4. *Wheat germ and brewer's yeast can supply some of the Vitamin B_{12} missing in a diet that does not include animal products.*
5. *Combining grains and beans in one meal produces a complete protein.*
6. *Homemade whole-grain bread is not only low in calories but can be made more nutritious by adding such ingredients as bran, soy milk, skim milk powder, and bone meal.*
7. *In order to make sure that the yogurt you eat is fresh, alive, and low in calories, you should make your own at home.*

8. *You can make a complete meal of a salad by adding cottage cheese, sunflower seeds, and fruit to a bowl of mixed vegetables.*

9. *An energy drink made of skim milk, protein powder, brewer's yeast, and fresh fruit can supply sufficient protein and carbohydrate for one meal.*

10. *High-protein drinks should not be substituted for more than one meal a day.*

6

How to Enrich
Macro-Nutrient Foods
for Safe, Rapid Weight Loss

Roberta R. had been fighting fat for years. "I have a hard time losing weight," she complained. "I'm always on a diet, but weight loss is slow, and I usually gain it back."

An analysis of Roberta's eating habits revealed that her diet was deficient in fiber. "My mother always told me not to eat anything I couldn't digest," she explained. "So I have always avoided coarse, indigestible foods." The solution to Roberta's problem was obvious. She needed more fiber—more of the type of foods she was avoiding. I told Roberta about the cellulose in raw fruits and vegetables, about the bran in whole-grain products, and how to *add* fiber to her foods. I told her all about fiber—everything I'm going to tell you in this chapter.

The result was that Roberta began to lose weight rapidly. She lost five to six pounds a week for several weeks. Weight loss then tapered down to two or three pounds a week. Over a period of 12 months, she lost more than 100 pounds of fat! "I had to buy all new clothes," Roberta noted with a sense of accomplishment, "but it was worth it. I threw away all my old clothes. I don't ever plan to wear an oversize dress again! I *know* the weight I've lost won't come back this time. I'm eating so well on my high-fiber diet that I plan to continue eating this way as long as I live."

The last time I saw Roberta, she was still slim and trim. "I

115

didn't tell you this before," she whispered, "but ever since I started that high-fiber diet, I haven't had any more trouble with my bowels."

You can benefit from a high-fiber macro-nutrient diet in many ways. Even when you no longer have any excess body fat to lose, you can use a high-fiber diet to improve your health.

THE MANY BENEFITS OF A HIGH-FIBER DIET

Research in recent years has revealed that adequate food fiber in the diet helps prevent such diseases as diverticulitis, colon cancer, hardened arteries, and hemorrhoids. Doctors believe that constipation resulting from low-fiber food residue forms tiny pressure pouches (diverticuli) in the walls of the colon. Fecal waste retained too long in the colon inflames these pouches and allows bacterial activity to convert bile acids to cancer-causing toxins. Furthermore, over consumption of such zero-fiber, high-fat foods as meat, dairy products, and processed carbohydrates may contribute to a buildup of fat and cholesterol in the blood. Straining to empty a clogged and tightly packed bowel swells rectal veins, resulting in painful hemorrhoids, and so on.

High-protein, high-fat diets not only deprive the bowels of healthful fiber but also supply saturated fats that might contribute to clogging of the arteries. Too much fat of any kind may contribute to the development of some forms of cancer. (Heart disease is presently the nation's No. 1 killer; cancer is No. 2. *Colon cancer* is the second most common cause of death from cancer.) Refined carbohydrates play a role in the development of diabetes, obesity, colon cancer, and other diseases.

Obviously, a major part of the solution to many health problems is found in use of a diet that stresses such fiber-rich natural carbohydrates as fresh fruits and vegetables and whole-grain products. A diet high in natural carbohydrates *is* a fiber-rich diet. This is one reason why the new U.S. Dietary Goals now recommend that Americans depend upon complex natural carbohydrates for at least 48 percent of their energy intake (58 percent if you exclude refined sugars), with 12 percent of energy supplied by protein and 30 percent by fat. If you follow these guidelines, you'll be able to control your body weight more effectively.

How to Increase Your Intake of Fiber

Fresh fruits, raw vegetables, and whole-grains all supply food fiber—and the more fiber in your diet the more weight you can lose. If you want to lose a little more weight a little faster, you can add some *extra* fiber to your diet in the form of miller's bran. Too much miller's bran might be harmful, however, so you'll have to use it cautiously. It's always best to get your fiber from natural foods whenever possible. Small amounts of miller's bran may then be added to selected foods. When your body weight is down to a desirable level, you can get all the fiber you need from a good high-fiber diet. Persons who are unable to eat properly should, of course, continue to use miller's bran as a supplement.

Types of Fiber

Fiber is generally divided into two categories: the less digestible *bran* fiber from grains and the more digestible *cellulose* fiber from fruits and vegetables. The cellulose or food fiber in fruits and vegetables can be broken down to release nutrients, especially in the case of cooked vegetables, but the fiber supplied by whole grains passes undigested through the intestinal tract in the form of silky fibers.

You need both types of fiber in your diet for good health, since both have different effects in your body. But they should be supplied in a balanced diet that includes some of *all* the basic foods. A diet too heavy in whole-grain products is not only unbalanced but may actually interfere with absorption of essential minerals. The phytates in the bran portion of whole grains, for example, tend to combine with iron, zinc, copper, magnesium, calcium, and chromium to reduce absorption of these minerals. This interference is not significant in a balanced diet that includes fiber-rich fruits and vegetables. (Since processed grains are *deficient* in minerals, you'll lose more minerals eating processed grains than you will eating whole grains that contain phytates. Besides, *cooking* grains diminishes their phytate content.) In an all-grain diet, however, deficiencies might result.

When large amounts of uncooked miller's bran are added to the diet to block absorption of calories, there is a definite danger of developing a mineral deficiency. This is one reason why I do not recommend a "bran diet" in which pure bran is substituted for a meal or eaten as a cereal. Using pure bran to speed weight loss by substituting bran for food is not worth the risk. It would be much better to add a small amount of bran to cereals, breads, yogurt, and other natural foods in a balanced diet. The additional bulk provided by the bran fiber should reduce calorie intake enough to result in loss of an extra half pound or so of body fat a week.

Reduce Blood Cholesterol with Food Fiber

In addition to reducing body fat, food fiber may also play a role in reducing blood cholesterol. We know that bile secreted into the intestine by the gall bladder is formed from cholesterol. Fiber in the intestine combines with bile salts which are then eliminated as waste. The greater the fiber intake the more bile produced and excreted and the lower the blood cholesterol. Some researchers say that all forms of fiber combine with bile salts. Others say that wheat bran does *not* combine with bile salts and that only the fiber of beans, the pectin of apples, and the hemicellulose provided by cereal grains can reduce blood cholesterol.

Vegetable fiber (cellulose) holds more water than wheat fiber (bran). Water-holding fiber produces healthful bulk for the intestinal tract. Vegetable fiber can be digested, however, and is less likely to reach the colon than bran. In fact, one researcher has estimated that 75 percent of the dietary fiber you consume disappears in its passage through the intestine because of the digestion of cellulose by intestinal bacteria. So you may have to depend more upon wheat bran than upon vegetable cellulose for the fiber you need for good colon function.

Obviously, there may be differences in opinion about the effects of different types of fiber in the diet. To be on the safe side, keep your diet *balanced* so that you get fiber from fruits and vegetables as well as from whole grains.

How Much Fiber Do You Need?

The total amount of fiber in the food you eat is known as *dietary fiber*. The indigestible portion of the fiber that reaches your colon is known as *crude fiber*. Wheat bran, for example, is a dietary fiber that yields about nine percent crude fiber (nine grams of fiber per 100 grams of bran). The cellulose in a raw carrot yields only about one percent crude fiber. Dietary fiber benefits your entire intestinal tract. Generally, however, only the crude fiber content of fecal (colon) waste is measured in judging fiber intake.

The diet of the average American supplies only about four grams of crude fiber a day. Some digestive specialists recommend that we consume at least as much fiber as Americans consumed back in the days when foods were not processed and when heart disease and cancer of the colon were rare.

No one knows for sure exactly how much fiber we need for the best of health. Dr. Neil Painter, a British cancer researcher, recommends 12 to 14 grams of crude fiber a day for adults. This amount of fiber can easily be supplied by natural foods. Studies of diets of rural Africans who rarely have colon cancer revealed that they consume an average of 23 grams of crude fiber a day, less than one ounce (28.35 grams per ounce). This is about six times more fiber than the average American consumes.

If you eat fresh fruits and vegetables and whole-grain products and eliminate refined and processed foods from your diet, you'll get all the fiber you need for good health. Two teaspoons of miller's bran added to each meal, however, would be helpful in a reducing diet.

In this chapter, I'll tell you how to increase the amount of fiber in your diet by eating natural foods and by adding miller's bran to your diet. Once you learn which foods are highest in fiber, you may simply increase your intake of these foods in balancing your diet. Then, for more rapid weight loss, you can add *extra* fiber to a high-fiber diet. It's important to make sure that you depend primarily upon *food* for most of your fiber. You may supplement your diet with miller's bran, but you should not substitute miller's bran for food.

Fiber Content of Popular Foods

When planning your meals for an increased intake of food fiber, it's enough to know that fresh fruits, vegetables, and whole-grain cereals and breads contain fiber, while meat, fish, poultry, dairy products, and processed foods do *not* contain fiber. Balancing your diet so that 58 percent of your energy intake is supplied by natural carbohydrate will automatically supply the fiber you need for good health. It would be helpful, however, to know which foods are highest in crude fiber when planning a high-fiber reducing diet.

How foods are prepared can have much to do with their fiber content. *Cooking fruits and vegetables, for example, diminishes their fiber content.* Overcooked vegetables may have very little fiber value. So remember what I told you in Chapter 4. *Eat your fruits raw and cook your vegetables as little as possible.* Grains should always be cooked to make them more digestible and to destroy their phytates. Fortunately, cooking a whole grain does not diminish its fiber value.

The crude fiber content of the basic foods varies considerably. Half a cup of all-bran cereal contains about three grams of fiber, while an equal amount of some other cereal might contain less than one gram of fiber. A slice of whole-wheat bread contains about half a gram of fiber. An apple with its skin supplies two grams of fiber, but a peach may contain only half a gram of fiber. Half a cup of brussels sprouts contains about two grams of fiber, twice as much fiber as half a cup of green beans. It may take a cup of sunflower seeds to equal the two grams of fiber in half a cup of nuts.

The Best Sources of Fiber

Pure bran is the richest source of fiber. Rice bran, for example, is about 11 percent fiber. Miller's bran is nine percent fiber. Among the foods, *whole-grain breads and cereals are the best sources of fiber.* Whole wheat, rye, pumpernickel, bran muffins, and corn bread are high-fiber breads. Shredded wheat, Grape Nuts, oats, wheat germ, puffed rice, buckwheat, bulgur, brown rice, and cracked wheat are good examples of high-fiber cereals. Bran cereal is highest in fiber (about 7.8 percent). If you enjoy popcorn, you'll be pleased to learn that plain popcorn is low in calories and high in fiber. Corn germ is about 18 percent fiber, and it does not contain the phytates found in wheat germ and bran. It's also a complete protein. When corn germ becomes more readily available, it will be a good fiber substitute for persons who are allergic to wheat gluten or who do not tolerate wheat too well.

Raw fruits and berries are good sources of fiber. Most raw berries contain more fiber than raw fruits. An apple, for example, is about one percent fiber. Blackberries, on the other hand, are about four percent fiber and raspberries about five percent fiber. So be sure to enclude boysenberries, blueberries, cranberries, loganberries, strawberries, and other fresh berries in your diet along with apples, oranges, bananas, figs, grapefruit, peaches, pears, pineapple, plums, and other raw fruits. Dried fruits are especially high in fiber (but high in sugar). A dried fig is about 5.6 percent fiber and dried apricots about 3.8 percent fiber. When you want a fiber-rich dessert, select a dried fruit.

Seeds, nuts, peas, and dried beans are also high-fiber foods. Chickpeas and soybeans are about five percent fiber. Sunflower seeds are about 3.8 percent fiber. Include all kinds of seeds and nuts in your diet, but remember that they are high in fat. All fresh and dried peas and beans are excellent sources of fiber.

Moisturize Your Colon with Vegetable Fiber

The cellulose fiber supplied by vegetables is especially helpful in holding water in your colon. Cooked turnips are about nine percent fiber if they are not overcooked. An artichoke is about 2.5 percent fiber. It's important to include a wide variety of vegetables in your diet—whatever is in season. You can't go wrong with such vegetables as asparagus, beets, broccoli, brussels sprouts, cabbage, carrots, cauliflower, celery, corn, chard, cucumber, eggplant, collards, kale, escarole, mustard, turnips, lettuce, okra, onions, parsley, potatoes, radishes, rutabagas, spinach, string beans, squash, tomatoes, and zucchini.

If you'd like to estimate your crude fiber intake in grams, refer to the food-fiber table in this chapter in selecting high-fiber fruits, vegetables, and grains (Table 6-1). Try to keep you fiber intake up around 15 grams a day.

Note: In one study of fiber, researchers found that subjects who consumed 16 grams of crude fiber a day for three weeks excreted significantly higher amounts of sodium, potassium, and magnesium than did control subjects. So don't go overboard on consumption of fiber. Keep your diet balanced with food selections from *all* the basic food groups.

Recommended reading: *Nutrition: Concepts and Controversies,* by Hamilton and Whitney, West Publishing Company, St. Paul, Minnesota.

Table 6-1

100 Grams (3.5 Ounces)   **Grams (Percent) of Fiber**

Almonds, dried	2.6
Apples with skin	1.0
Apples, dried	3.1
Apricots, raw	.6
Apricots, dried	3.0
Artichokes, raw or cooked	2.4
Asparagus, raw or cooked	.7
Avocados	1.6
Bananas, raw	.5
Bananas, dried	2.0
Barley, dark	.9
Beans, common, cooked	1.5
Beans, lima, cooked	1.8
Beans, mung, cooked	.7
Beans, snap, cooked	1.0
Beets, red, raw or cooked	.8
Beet greens, cooked	1.1
Blackberries (including dewberries, boysenberries, and youngberries) raw	4.1
Blueberries, raw	1.5
Bran flakes (40 percent bran)	3.6
Brazil nuts	3.1
Breads:	
Cracked wheat	.5
American rye	.4
Pumpernickel	1.1
Whole wheat	1.6
Broadbeans, mature, raw, dry	6.7
Broccoli, raw or cooked	1.5
Brussels sprouts, raw or cooked	1.6
Buckwheat, whole grain	9.9
Buckwheat flour, dark	1.6
Bulgur (parboiled wheat)	1.7
Cabbage, raw or cooked	.8
Carob flour	7.7
Carrots, raw or cooked	1.0
Cashew nuts	1.4
Cauliflower, raw or cooked	1.0
Celery, raw or cooked	.6
Chard, Swiss, raw	.8
Cherries, raw, sweet	.4
Chestnuts, fresh	1.1
Chestnuts, dried	2.5
Chestnut flour	2.0
Chickpeas (garbanzos), raw, dry	5.0
Chives, raw	1.1
Coconut meat, fresh	4.0
Collards, leaves	1.2

Table 6-1 (continued)

100 Grams (3.5 Ounces)   **Grams (Percent) of Fiber**

Corn, field, whole grain, raw	2.0
Corn flour	.7
Corn grits, cooked	.1
Corn flakes	.7
Corn pone, whole grain	.8
Cornmeal, whole ground, unbolted	1.6
Cowpeas (including blackeye peas), dry, cooked	1.0
Cranberries, raw	1.4
Cucumbers, unpeeled	.6
Dandelion greens, raw	1.6
Dates, domestic	2.3
Eggplant, raw or cooked	.9
Elderberries, raw	7.0
Endive, raw	.9
Figs, raw	1.2
Figs, dried	5.6
Filberts (hazelnuts)	3.0
Gooseberries, raw	1.9
Grapefruit	.2
Grapes, raw	.6
Groundcherries, raw	2.8
Guavas, common, raw	5.6
Guavas, strawberry, raw	6.4
Horseradish, raw	2.4
Hyacinth beans, dry, raw	6.9
Jerusalem artichoke, raw	.8
Kale, leaves with stems, raw	1.3
Kohlrabi, raw	1.0
Kumquats, raw	3.7
Lentiles, dry, cooked	1.2
Lettuce, raw	.7
Loganberries, raw	3.0
Macadamia nuts	2.5
Mangos, raw	.9
Millet, whole grain	3.2
Muffins, bran	1.8
Mushrooms, raw	.8
Muskmelon, honeydew, raw	.6
Mustard greens, cooked	.9
Mustard spinach, raw	1.0
Oatmeal, dry	1.2
Oatmeal, cooked	.2
Okra, cooked	.6
Olives, green	6.4
Onions, raw	.6
Oranges, peeled	.6
Papayas, raw	.9
Parsley, raw	1.5

Table 6-1 (continued)

100 Grams (3.5 Ounces)   **Grams (Percent) of Fiber**

Parsnips, raw	2.0
Peaches, raw	.6
Peaches, dried	3.1
Peanuts with skins, raw	2.4
Peanut flour, defatted	2.7
Pears with skin, raw	1.4
Peas, cooked	1.2
Peas, green, cooked	2.0
Pecans	2.3
Persimmons, raw	1.5
Pigeonpeas, raw, dry	7.0
Pineapple, raw	.4
Plums, hybrid, raw	.6
Popcorn, plain	2.2
Potatoes, baked in skin	.6
Potato flour	1.6
Prunes, dried, uncooked	1.6
Pumpkin, canned	1.3
Radishes, raw	.7
Raisins	.9
Raspberries, black, raw	5.1
Rhubarb, cooked	.6
Rice, brown, cooked	.3
Rice bran	11.5
Rutabagas, raw or cooked	1.1
Rye, whole grain	2.0
Rye flour, dark	2.4
Safflower seed meal	7.4
Seaweed, kelp, raw	6.8
Sesame seeds, whole, dry	6.3
Soybeans, dry, cooked	1.6
Soybean sprouts, cooked	.8
Soybean flour, low fat	2.5
Spinach, raw or cooked	.6
Squash, summer, raw or cooked	.6
Squash, winter, baked	1.8
Strawberries, raw	1.3
Sunflower seeds, dry	3.8
Sunflower seed flour	4.6
Sweet potatoes, baked in skin	.9
Tangerines, raw	.5
Tomatoes, raw	.5
Turnips, raw or cooked	.9
Turnip greens, cooked	.7
Walnuts, English	2.1
Water chestnut, raw	.8
Watercress, raw	.7

Table 6-1 (continued)

100 Grams (3.5 Ounces)	Grams (Percent) of Fiber
Watermelon	.3
Wheat, whole grain	2.3
Wheat flour, whole	2.3
Wheat bran, crude	9.1
Wheat germ, crude	2.5
Wheat cereal, whole, dry	2.2
Wheat germ, toasted	1.7
Wheat, puffed	2.0
Wheat, shredded	2.3
Wild rice, raw	1.0
Yam, raw	.9
Yeast, brewer's	1.7
Yeast, torula	3.3

CRUDE FIBER CONTENT OF FOOD SERVINGS*

The average food serving is about 100 grams (3.5 ounces) in weight. Grams of fiber per 100-gram portion of a food also represents the *percentage* of fiber. A quick look at these figures will quickly tell you which foods are highest in crude fiber. You'll notice, for example, that berries are especially high in fiber. Remember that meats and dairy products do not contain fiber and are therefore not listed.

More recent analysis of foods may show a higher crude fiber content than figures given in *Composition of Foods* and other government publications. But once you get the general idea, you won't have any trouble increasing your fiber intake in a balanced diet.

SELECTING AND PREPARING FIBER-RICH FOODS

Since fresh fruits, vegetables, and whole-grain products are fiber-rich carbohydrates, a balanced diet that stresses natural carbohydrates will normally provide adequate fiber. The more fiber in your diet, however, the easier it is to lose weight. So it might be a good idea to select the carbohydrates that contain the most fiber.

---

*Adapted from *Composition of Foods*, Agriculture Handbook No. 8, U.S. Department of Agriculture, Washington, D.C., Reprinted 1975.

When you select bread, for example, get the coarsest whole-grain bread you can find. I particularly enjoy eating wheat bread that contains whole wheat kernels or "berries." Such bread is chewy, tasty, and filling, and it provides fewer calories than white bread. One study revealed that 96 percent of the calories in white bread are absorbed compared with only 87 percent in the case of whole-grain bread. (See Chapter 5 for a high-fiber bread recipe.)

How to Lose 18 Pounds in Two Months by Eating Bread

The August, 1979, issue of the *American Journal of Clinical Nutrition* reported on an experiment in which overweight college students lost an average of 18 pounds in two months by adding 12 slices of a special fiber-rich bread to a daily low-calorie diet. The fiber content of the bread was increased to *two grams per slice* by adding cellulose (sawdust) to the bread dough. (A slice of whole wheat bread normally contains about half a gram of fiber, while a slice of white bread contains only one-tenth of one gram of fiber.)

You can increase the fiber content of the bread you eat by making your own and adding miller's bran. The cellulose of sawdust might be free of mineral-binding phytates, but I would still prefer the fiber supplied by bran. Eating fiber-rich bread early in a meal will provide satisfying bulk that will quickly satisfy your appetite so that less food is eaten.

Fiber in bread, in addition to acting as a mechanical barrier to absorption of calories, displaces energy nutrients with indigestible matter. Fiber also speeds the movement of food through the digestive tract, allowing less time for absorption of calories.

A Recipe for Fiber-Rich Corn Pone

My wife, Martha, often makes corn pone from fiber-rich medium ground whole corn. She adds sesame seeds to the cornmeal to form a complete protein as well as to add fiber. Such coarse bread is not fattening and can provide a real taste treat, especially when served with turnips, collards, and other fiber-rich greens. Here is Martha's recipe for old-fashioned corn pone:

3 cups white cornmeal
⅓ cup sesame seeds
½ teaspoon salt
¼ cup corn oil
Several cups of boiling water

Mix the meal, sesame seeds, and the salt. Pour in the corn oil and the water. Mix and form into patties. Bake in an oven for 50 minutes at 350 degrees Fahrenheit.

Keep Your Cereals Natural

Simply substituting whole-grain breads and cereals for their refined counterparts will add fiber as well as nutrients to your diet. Be sure to read the labels on the products you buy, however. Wheat cereals, for example, should be *100 percent whole wheat*, and they should not contain sugar or other sweeteners. Some refined cereals contain more sugar than anything else—and no bran at all!

Shredded wheat, oats, Grape Nuts, cracked wheat, bran flakes, and bulgur are good examples of whole-grain, sugar-free cereals. Granola is a popular whole-grain cereal that's high in fiber, but some commercial varieties tend to be high in calories. According to *Dietary Goals*, "Granola does have *slightly* more protein, calcium, riboflavin and niacin than plain cereals, but the difference is not great enough to make this a special reason for buying it. Its major disadvantages are its high calorie value, its high fat content, the high saturation of fat in the shredded coconut and its high cost."

I, personally, find most grocery store granola too sweet. So I usually mix it with shredded wheat, miller's bran, and diced fresh fruit. Sometimes I throw in a few sunflower seeds.

How to Make Granola at Home

You can make your own granola and keep sugar and fat at a minimum. Here's a recipe for a high-fiber granola that can be used as a cereal, as a snack, or as a topping for yogurt.

6 cups rolled oats
1 cup wheat germ
½ cup miller's bran
½ cup sesame seeds
½ cup sunflower seeds
1 cup chopped nuts
¼ cup slivered almonds
⅓ cup honey
⅓ cup vegetable oil
1 cup raisins
½ cup chopped dried apple

Mix the oats, wheat germ, bran, seeds, and nuts in a large bowl. Mix the honey and oil in a separate bowl and then mix the liquid into the dry ingredients. Spread the entire mixture over a large cookie sheet and bake at 300 degrees Fahrenheit for about half an hour. Stir frequently for even browning. Add the raisins and the chopped apple after the granola has cooled.

How to Conserve the Fiber of Vegetables

Cooking or steaming vegetables only slightly will preserve taste and nutrients as well as fiber. You can further increase the amount of fiber in your diet by eating vegetables raw and by cooking *fresh* vegetables so that you can include skins, strings, stems, outer leaves, and other portions of vegetables that cooks often throw out.

Coarse leafy vegetables such as spinach can be mixed into raw salads. Remember, however, that cutting or chopping greens results in loss of nutrients. For this reason, salad greens should be served whole or torn into large pieces by hand. The salad may then be cut as it is eaten.

If you eat your fruits raw, cook your vegetables as little as possible, and include whole-grain products in your meals, you'll have a high-fiber diet that is nutritious and simple to prepare. Best of all, you'll experience the *real taste* of food.

How to Add Fiber to Foods

There are many ways to increase the fiber in your diet. For example, oats, wheat germ, or bran can replace bread crumbs in recipes. Whole-grain flours can be used instead of white flour, whether you're baking cookies or making bread. Brown rice should *always* be selected over white rice when you have a choice. When fresh beans aren't available, dried peas or beans are always better than canned beans. Powdered potatoes should *never* be substituted for fresh, unpeeled potatoes. When you cook with tomatoes, use *fresh* tomatoes instead of canned tomatoes so that you can include the skins.

With a little imagination, you can think of many ways to increase the fiber in your diet. You can also add miller's bran to cooked and uncooked foods for extra fiber.

How to Use Miller's Bran as a Supplement

Generally, about two teaspoons of unprocessed miller's bran added to each meal will be enough to supplement a good reducing diet. You may either sprinkle the bran over foods or you may mix it into foods that must be cooked. Although miller's bran is referred to as "roughage," it's actually soft and silky in the intestinal tract. So there is no danger of intestinal irritation. The fiber in miller's bran simply provides water-holding bulk that improves intestinal function and reduces your appetite for other foods.

Since bran can interfere with absorption of minerals as well as calories, you must use bran as a supplement and not as a substitute for food. The trick is to add just enough miller's bran to your diet to reduce your calorie intake without creating a mineral deficiency.

Adding large, unaccustomed amounts of bran to your diet might result in abdominal distension and flatus (gas) because of the osmotic effect of bran. These problems usually disappear in four to six weeks. You can avoid such problems by increasing your intake of bran slowly over a period of time—up to about 25 grams a day.

When your stools are regular, moist, firm, and well-formed, you probably have adequate fiber in your diet.

Bran for Breakfast, Lunch, and Dinner

The best way to add fiber to your breakfast is to add bran to your cereal. A couple of teaspoons of miller's bran can be added to cold, uncooked cereal or to hot, cooked cereal. In either case, the bran will add a pleasant, chewy wheat flavor. I enjoy miller's bran on oatmeal just as well as on shredded wheat.

Don't buy instant or quick-cooking cereals, even if you plan to enrich them with miller's bran. In addition to being deficient in fiber, quick-cooking cereals may be deficient in vitamins and minerals.

Bran may also be added to soups, casseroles, dips, salads, sauces, meat loaf, homemade bread, and other foods. Some people stir bran into tomato juice and other beverages for an appetite-killing drink before meals. The bran swells in the stomach to produce a sensation of fullness that reduces desire for food.

Two teaspoons of bran mixed into a cup of yogurt is a filling, low-calorie snack. Try a spoonful of bran sprinkled over a baked apple if you need a natural laxative.

If you have pancakes for breakfast, make them with buckwheat or some other whole-grain flour that has been enriched with bran. Muffins prepared with miller's bran can replace bread, rolls, and biscuits.

Here's a good recipe for bran muffins:

1 cup unprocessed miller's bran or bran cereal
1 cup whole wheat flour
1 teaspoon salt
1 teaspoon cinnamon
2 tablespoons vegetable oil
1 cup skim milk
4 eggs (separated)
3 tablespoons honey
½ cup raisins

Mix the bran, flour, salt, and cinnamon. In another bowl, combine oil, milk, raisins, beaten egg yolks, and honey; add this to the flour mixture. Beat the egg whites stiff and fold into the batter. Bake in oiled muffin tins at 375 degrees Fahrenheit for 30 minutes.

A Single Remedy for Overweight and Irregularity

Bran-supplemented foods in a balanced diet that includes fresh fruits, vegetables, and whole-grain products will help regulate your intestinal tract as well as keep your body lean. One patient who added miller's bran to her diet in order to correct an elimination problem lost nearly 60 pounds of body fat in a year. "I went from a size 18 dress to a size 12," she said. "And I never did have to take another laxative. I still add two teaspoons of bran to a cup of plain yogurt twice a day.

Don't Forget Desserts!

You should avoid cooked desserts as much as possible if you are overweight. Commercial sweets should be avoided altogether. When you do prepare a cooked dessert, it would be better to whip up a whole-grain sweet rather than a sugary, white-flour product. Cookies, cakes, fruit pies, and puddings made at home, for example, can be enriched with miller's bran so that they contribute fiber with a minimum number of calories. Substituting half a cup of wheat germ or bran for half a cup of flour will boost the fiber content of pie crust and other pastries. *Whole-grain flour can be used instead of processed flour.*

Bran can be substituted for a portion of the Graham crackers used in making pie shells. You can mix bran with cinnamon, margarine, and a little brown sugar for use as a topping on fruit desserts—but only on special occasions! Plain wheat germ makes an excellent topping on yogurt or ice cream.

Plain fresh fruits and dried fruits make good high-fiber desserts. It's not likely that you'll eat an excessive amount of fresh fruit, since your appetite mechanism will usually register satisfaction very quickly. Cooked desserts, on the other hand, may artificially stimulate your appetite, making it difficult to quit eating. So try to select fresh fruits for dessert whenever you have a choice—at least most of the time.

How to Make Bran Brownies

You can find many good recipes for wholesome desserts in natural food cookbooks. In the meantime, here's a recipe for bran brownies that will satisfy anyone's sweet tooth:

2 squares unsweetened chocolate
⅓ cup margarine
½ cup honey
1 teaspoon vanilla
⅔ cup sifted unbleached flour
2 tablespoons instant coffee powder
½ teaspoon baking powder
½ teaspoon salt
2 tablespoons wheat germ
2 eggs
½ cup bran or bran cereal
½ cup chopped nuts

*Melt the chocolate and the margarine together and then stir in
the honey and the vanilla. Mix the flour, coffee, salt, baking
powder, and wheat germ together and then blend with chocolate mixture. Beat in eggs, one at a time. Fold in bran and
nuts. Spread in 9 × 9 × 2-inch baking pan and bake at 350
degrees Fahrenheit for 30 minutes. Cool and cut into 12
brownies.*

A Recipe for Carob Carrot Bran Cake

Try this recipe for a fiber-rich cake that's not overly sweet:

*½ cup rasins
¾ cup whole wheat flour
¼ cup soy flour
½ cup bran flakes
3 tablespoons carob flour
1½ teaspoon cinnamon
2 teaspoons grated orange or lemon rind
¼ teaspoon salt
1 cup grated carrots
2 eggs, separated*

*Put the rasins in a cup and add hot water until the cup is full.
Pour the contents of the cup into a bowl and add the remaining
ingredients except for the egg whites. Beat the egg whites until
they are stiff and fold into the mixture in the bowl. Place in an
oiled bread pan and bake at 350 degrees Fahrenheit for about
55 minutes. Delicious with yogurt!*

SUMMARY

1. *Adequate fiber in your diet helps prevent disease as well as overweight.*
2. *Complex (natural) carbohydrates such as fresh fruits, vegetables,
   and whole-grain products are the best sources of food fiber.*
3. *Cooking fruits and vegetables diminishes their fiber value by destroying their cellulose.*
4. *Cooking whole grains reduces harmful phytates but does not destroy
   their bran fiber.*
5. *Miller's bran can be used as a supplement to speed weight loss by
   providing fiber that interferes with absorption of calories.*
6. *Remember that an excessive amount of miller's bran in the diet might
   reduce absorption of essential minerals.*

7. *Two heaping teaspoons of miller's bran added to each meal will be about right for persons on a reducing diet.*
8. *Always buy* whole-grain *cereals that do not contain sugar or any other sweetener.*
9. *Wheat germ and miller's bran (or bran cereals) can be mixed into such dishes as meat loaf, muffins, and casseroles* before *cooking them.*
10. *If you must have cooked desserts, prepare whole-grain sweets that can be enriched with bran.*

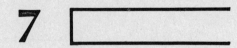

7

How to Nibble
on Macro-Nutrient Foods
for Pleasurable Slimming

Eat all you want and still lose weight! How many times have you seen this statement used in the promotion of a reducing diet? Some diets maintain that you can eat all you want of almost *anything* and still lose weight. Of course, there's no healthful way to stuff yourself and lose body fat as a result. If you get your energy nutrients from protein, carbohydrate, and fat in a balanced diet as you are supposed to do, you'll have to limit your food intake to keep your calorie intake down. With 48 to 58 percent of your energy intake coming from natural carbohydrates, however, you can eat generously enough to divide your food intake into five or six small meals a day.

The greater the percentage of fresh vegetables in your diet the more you can eat without exceeding your calorie needs. Strict vegetarians must eat large amounts of vegetables to get adequate protein—and they can do so without getting fat because vegetables are low in calories. But a diet consisting solely of vegetables is not a balanced diet and is therefore not a healthful diet.

Such dietary fads as neutralizing stomach acid with alkalizers in order to interfere with the digestion of large amounts of food, or stuffing yourself with bran to prevent absorption of calories, can only result in bad health along with loss of body weight. So don't fall for oddball diets that do not attach importance to calorie intake.

If you take in more calories each day than you burn, you'll gain weight. It's as simple as that. If you don't absorb an adequate number of calories, you won't absorb adequate nutrients. What you must do is eat foods that supply nutrients with as few calories as possible. You can do this by controlling your calorie intake on a balanced diet of natural foods. This will enable you to control your reducing power pedal very effectively. Furthermore, if you eat *high-fiber* natural foods, you won't absorb all the calories you consume. This is one reason why you can eat generous amounts of natural foods without getting fat. As you know from reading Chapter 2, fiber-rich natural carbohydrates provide the best available fuel for your fat-burner throttle.

If your diet is balanced, it won't be necessary to eat large amounts of food to get the nutrients you need. But if you eat the right foods, you *can* nibble!

I told you in the opening chapters of this book how to divide your energy nutrients among carbohydrate, protein, and fat foods so that you can control your calorie intake and stay healthy. There are occasions, however, when nibbling can be beneficial. Persons suffering from blood sugar problems, for example, must nibble between meals to keep their appetite under control.

Actor Joseph Campanella has discovered that a good diet and an active schedule allows him to snack without gaining weight. "I like to snack on Italian cheeses," he admitted in a personal interview, "sometimes a bowl of cold cereal, such as granola. We eat fresh fruit every night."

Lyle Waggoner of TV's "Wonder Woman" keeps his weight down by snacking on simple foods. "I like to snack a lot," he says. "So I have four, five, or six small meals a day." At six feet four inches and 200 pounds, Lyle looks great!

FOUR METHODS OF NIBBLING

There are at least four ways to nibble on a healthful reducing diet.

1. You can figure your calorie needs according to your weight goal (see Chapter 3) and then divide your allowable food intake into five or six small meals a day. If you exclude all processed foods and get most of your energy from natural carbohydrates, your food intake will be large enough to allow nibbling between meals.

Harold T. felt that eating three large meals a day caused sluggishness by overfilling his stomach. So he chose to eat five small meals a day. "Eating smaller amounts of food more frequently, I'm better able to concentrate on my work," Harold observed. "And I'm actually losing more weight than I did previously. For example, I lost three pounds last week instead of the usual pound or two."

2. Raw vegetables are so rich in food fiber and so low in calories that you can eat all you want of your favorite raw vegetable between meals as long as you include other basic foods in your regular meals. Nibbling on raw vegetables should, however, reduce your appetite at mealtime.

Marsha D. kept all kinds of fresh vegetables in her refrigerator. Everytime she felt an urge to eat something, she nibbled on a carrot, a piece of celery, a section of cucumber, or some other favorite vegetable. The result was that she ate smaller portions during regular meals. Adding up her total weekly calorie intake revealed that she was taking in about 3,500 fewer calories than she needed to maintain her existing weight. So she lost a pound a week by doing nothing more than eating raw vegetables between meals.

3. If you suffer from hypoglycemia, or low blood sugar, you can best keep your blood sugar up by snacking on such low-fat protein foods as toasted soybeans and yogurt. You must then eat less at mealtime to keep your calorie intake within limits.

Lynn T. complained of fatigue and a craving for sweets. She was advised to include a protein-rich between-meal snack in her diet. Whatever she ate—chicken, cheese, nuts, or skim milk products—was deducted from her calorie allowance at mealtime. Her craving for sweets disappeared, her fatigue vanished, and her weight loss proceeded as usual. "I'm still losing three or four pounds a week," Lynn reported with obvious satisfaction. "And I'm much more alert and energetic."

4. Another way to eat between meals is to eat something bulky and non-nutritious simply to kill your appetite by filling your stomach. Bran supplements, or bran added to a low-calorie snack such as yogurt, for example, can be filling and satisfying. Since bran interferes with absorption of nutrients, large amounts of bran should not be taken with regular meals. Between meals, however, you may use bran to fill your stomach with water-holding, zero-calorie bulk.

Nina L. wanted to lose five or six pounds a week for a few weeks without suffering from the hunger pangs of an empty stomach. So, in addition to adding miller's bran to her breakfast cereal, she ate milk-moistened bran between meals and then ate less at mealtime. "I lost 15 pounds in three weeks," Nina reported. "I've never lost so much weight so fast!" Since Nina had only a few more pounds to lose, I advised her to switch to a simple 1,500-calorie diet to guard against a nutritional deficiency. In another month or so, she reached her ideal weight. "I'm so pleased with the way I look now that I won't ever let myself get fat again," Nina vowed.

No one has to tolerate a fat body. Any one of the many tips outlined in this book may provide you with the key to successful dieting.

Pick the Nibbling Method Best Suited for You

I'll discuss the nibbling methods in more detail in the remaining portion of this chapter. You can pick the method that best suits your needs. The one thing that all these methods have in common is that they call for basic foods that are high in fiber. These foods won't displace the nutrients and the calories you need for good health. In fact, you can nibble to contribute to your intake of nutrients so that you can eat smaller meals. Or you can nibble to make it easier to avoid exceeding your recommended calorie intake at mealtime.

Remember that there is no secret nibbling diet or some undiscovered short-term diet that can guarantee permanent weight loss. *Successful dieting means following general rules that govern your eating habits every day of your life.* If you do not know how to eat properly, or if you do not know why you should or should not eat certain types of foods, no diet will keep you slim. So if you're going to nibble, you should do so with at least a modicum of knowledge of the foods you eat.

You'll have an adequate knowledge of nutrition when you finish reading this book. Once you get the basic idea, you won't have to follow a specific diet. This is one reason why you should read this entire book rather than simply follow a copied 1,200-calorie diet. No diet will work for you very long if you do not know *how* to diet.

1. HOW TO EAT SIX TIMES A DAY
AND STILL LOSE WEIGHT

I rarely eat between meals. There is some evidence to indicate, however, that you might actually take in *fewer* calories if you eat four or five small meals a day rather than one or two big meals. One reason for this is that a between-meal snack takes the edge off your appetite so that you don't overeat at mealtime. Also, smaller meals do not force storage of body fat by overloading your blood with glucose and fat.

It's essential that snacks consist of natural, low-calorie foods that are rich in water and fiber. Fresh fruits, for example, make a good between-meal snack. So do raw vegetables. You should *never* snack on doughnuts, candy, soft drinks, and other processed foods. In addition to providing calories without fiber, processed snacks may artificially stimulate your appetite. Once you start snacking on chips, crackers, salted nuts, pretzels, and other commercial snacks, you might not be able to stop. As the TV ad says, "You can't eat just one!"

Plan Your Nibbling According to Your Calorie Needs

Turn back to Chapter 3 and use the calculations in that chapter to determine your calorie needs according to calories per pound of ideal bodyweight. If you're still in the process of reducing your body weight, your calorie intake should be *less* than what you need to maintain your ideal weight. For example, if you are overweight and you want to lose two pounds a week, you should be taking in 1,000 fewer calories a day than you would need to maintain your projected ideal weight.

Remember that 48 percent of your energy intake should come from natural carbohydrates and about 22 percent from protein. Once you determine which foods you should be eating to take in the recommended number of calories (with the correct percentage of energy nutrients), you simply divide those foods into three meals and three snacks.

If you are *maintaining* your ideal weight, you simply limit your daily calorie intake to the number of calories required to maintain that weight. With a larger food intake on a maintenance diet, you'll get adequate protein with 58 percent of your energy nutrients coming from natural carbohydrates and only 12 percent from protein.

The average reducing diet will call for about 1,500 calories a day, while the average maintenance diet might call for 2,500 calories a day (15 calories per pound of existing weight).

A Quick Review

Suppose you're overweight and you *should* weigh 140 pounds. If you are fairly active and you already weighed 140 pounds, you'd have to take in 2,100 calories a day to *maintain* that weight. In order to burn stored body fat to *reduce* your weight to 140 pounds, you'd have to take in *fewer* than 2,100 calories a day. Since one pound of body fat contains 3,500 calories, you'd have to create a calorie deficit of 500 calories a day to lose one pound a week. A deficit of 1,000 calories a day would result in loss of *two* pounds a week. This means that in order to lose two pounds a week, you'd have to limit your daily calorie intake to 1,100 calories a day. When your weight is down to 140 pounds, you may then increase your calorie intake to 2,100 calories a day.

Obviously, if you want to nibble between meals, you must do so within your calorie requirement. And you must be sure to figure your calorie requirement according to the *average* ideal weight for a person of your height and frame. So be sure to use the height-weight chart in Chapter 3. Don't try to reach a weight goal that is not appropriate for you.

Dividing a 1,200-Calorie Reducing Diet into Three Meals and Three Snacks

In Chapter 2, I outlined a 1,200+ calorie diet that supplies all the energy nutrients in the correct proportions. You can divide such a diet into meals and snacks in any manner you like. It doesn't matter whether you eat your eggs at breakfast or at dinner, for example, as long as you include all the recommended foods in the course of a day. Just make sure you have a complete protein in each meal (see Chapter 5).

Here's how I'd divide up a 1,200-calorie diet:

Breakfast

2 shredded wheat biscuits
1 cup skim milk
1 large egg
1 cup unsweetened coffee

Mid-Morning Snack

1 orange

Lunch

3 ounces broiled fish or chicken
1 stalk cooked broccoli
½ cup cooked carrots
1 slice whole-wheat bread with one pat of butter
Water or unsweetened tea

Mid-Afternoon Snack

1 peach

Dinner

½ cup cooked carrots
1 cup cooked cabbage
1 baked potato with one tablespoon vegetable oil
1 slice whole-wheat bread
1 cup skim milk

Evening Snack

1 apple

If you feel that you are not getting enough to eat on the above diet, eliminate the tablespoon of vegetable oil (125 calories) and substitute raw fruit and vegetables. An apple or an orange supplies about 70 calories. A raw carrot supplies 20 calories, and a stalk of raw celery only five calories. It would take 25 stalks of celery to supply 125 calories!

When you eat fruit, be sure to eat the *whole* fruit. Don't squeeze out the juice and throw away the pulp. It's the *fiber* in raw fruit that makes it a good low-calorie snack.

See Chapter 10 for a maintenance diet that supplies 2,000 calories or more. If you stick to fresh, natural foods as I have suggested throughout this book, you'll be able to eat well and maintain your body weight. In fact, if your diet is balanced so that 58 percent of your energy intake comes from natural carbohydrates, it would take a large amount of food to supply the 2,500 or so calories you'd need on a maintenance diet. This means that you can just about nibble to your heart's content if you stick to the recommended foods.

2. HOW TO KILL YOUR APPETITE BY NIBBLING ON RAW VEGETABLES

Persons who habitually or compulsively nibble between meals may have to limit their nibbling to raw vegetables to order to avoid an oversupply of calories. One of the secrets of successful, *healthful* dieting is to eat a balanced diet but to eat *less* than usual at mealtime. You can do this more effectively if you nibble on low-calorie, fiber-rich vegetables between meals to reduce your appetite by filling your stomach with fiber.

You may eat all the raw vegetables you want between meals. Then, at mealtime, you eat only as much as necessary to satisfy your appetite. To get the nutrients you need for good health, however, you should be sure to balance each meal with the basic foods. If your foods are fresh and natural, your appetite mechanism will keep your calorie intake down at a level that's best for you. Write down everything you eat during the day so that you can measure your calorie intake against the Table of Nutritive Values in Chapter 12.

Suggestions for Vegetable Snacks

You can snack on practically any raw vegetable except peas and beans. Carrots, cauliflower buds, zucchini, celery, cucumbers, lettuce, tomatoes, radishes, onions, broccoli flowerets, bell pepper, sweet potatoes, squash, cabbage, and other vegetables, for example, can be sliced, diced, or cut into sticks for convenient snacking. Pick the vegetables you like best. If you like, you can dip your vegetables into yogurt laced with bran and lemon juice or flavored with cinnamon, nutmeg, or vanilla.

Popcorn is a great low-calorie snack. One cup of unbuttered popcorn contains only 25 calories.

All raw vegetables are low in calories. One carrot, for example, supplies only about 20 calories, one cup of cauliflower buds 25 calories, one stalk of celery 5 calories, one peeled cucumber 30 calories, two large lettuce leaves 10 calories, one-half tomato 20 calories, four radishes 5 calories, and one onion 40 calories.

You don't have to worry about eating too many raw vegetables—at least as far as calories are concerned. The fiber and the water content of vegetables are so high that you simply cannot eat enough raw vegetables to build up body fat. Yet, the bulk supplied by vegetables will reduce your appetite at mealtime. Be sure to chew raw vegetables thoroughly, lest you suffer indigestion. Persons who have difficulty chewing or digesting raw vegetables might prefer to liquefy them in a blender.

If you don't enjoy the taste of raw vegetables, use a dip to add flavor. This will add a few calories, but not enough to hurt. Plain yogurt, with or without lemon juice, makes a tasty dip. Or you can mix a more elaborate dip.

Recipe for a Yogurt Dip

> *1 medium cucumber, peeled*
> *1½ cups low-fat yogurt*
> *½ teaspoon salt*
> *1 tablespoon chopped chives or onions*
> *¼ teaspoon dried mint*
> *¼ teaspoon black pepper*
> *Dash Worcestershire sauce*
>
> *Mix the cucumber with one-half cup yogurt in a blender and then mix in remaining ingredients. Refrigerate for a few hours before using. One tablespoon supplies about nine calories.*

A Between-Meal Salad

You might prefer to mix raw, cut vegetables to make a salad for between-meal snacks. You can use lemon juice, vinegar, yogurt, or a mixture of lemon juice and yogurt as a dressing. You may also mix in a little miller's bran for additional fiber if you like.

Since you are allowed up to two tablespoons of fat in a balanced low-calorie diet, you may mix vegetable oil into a homemade

Italian dressing. If you do, you should eliminate fat servings (butter and oil) in your meals.

A Recipe for Italian Dressing

2 tablespoons vegetable oil
2 teaspoons red wine vinegar
⅛ teaspoons each of basil and oregano (leaves)
Salt and pepper to taste

All of these ingredients combined will provide enough dressing for a midmorning and midafternoon salad snack. (One tablespoon of vegetable oil supplies about 125 calories.)

3. HOW TO CONTROL LOW BLOOD SUGAR
BY EATING BETWEEN MEALS

Hypoglycemia, or low blood sugar, was once a rare disorder. Today, because of excessive consumption of sugar, white flour, and other refined carbohydrates, hypoglycemia is becoming more common. The reason for this is easily explained. We all know that the pancreas produces insulin to convert blood sugar to glycogen for storage and for use as energy. When you eat fresh, natural foods, your sugar intake is low. Also, the sugar (glucose) provided by natural foods is absorbed slowly in small amounts. But when you eat *refined* carbohydrates, large amounts of glucose are quickly absorbed. This results in a sudden and excessive rise in blood sugar. The pancreas is compelled to act quickly in restoring the blood sugar level to normal.

Years of abusing or overworking the pancreas by eating excessive amounts of refined carbohydrates results in a pancreatic hypersensitivity. The pancreas then overreacts every time refined carbohydrates are eaten, forcing removal of an excessive amount of glucose from the blood. This results in weakness, shakiness, mental confusion, a craving for sweets, and other symptoms. (Remember that your brain cells as well as your muscles use glucose for fuel. When glucose is forcibly removed from your blood as a result of a pancreatic reaction, it is stored as glycogen and fat, thus reducing the amount of fuel available for immediate use by your body.)

If you suffer from true pancreatic hypersensitivity, you'll experience symptoms of hypoglycemia two to four hours after eating a refined carbohydrate. The hunger that results may lead to an irresistible urge to eat something sweet. This can lead to the development of diabetes (pancreatic exhaustion) as well as to overweight. Diabetes is already the seventh leading cause of death in the United States, and projections indicate that the number of diabetics in this country will *double* in the next 15 years! Obesity is also one of the nation's leading health problems. And obesity, like hypoglycemia, is often the forerunner of serious health problems.

Obviously, you should avoid excessive consumption of refined carbohydrates in order to protect your health as well as to control your body weight. Unlike refined carbohydrates, *natural* carbohydrates do *not* lead to the development of hypoglycemia, obesity, and diabetes. In fact, as you learned in earlier chapters of this book, the high-fiber content of natural carbohydrates makes them less fattening than other types of foods. And there is evidence to show that a diet high in complex (natural) carbohydrates is actually helpful in the *treatment* of diabetes *(Dietary Goals)*.

The Problem of Diagnosis

Although hypoglycemia is becoming increasingly common, it has become a catchall diagnosis by practitioners who peddle nutritional supplements on the basis of urinalysis, hair analysis, and other unorthodox tests. So check with your doctor. Don't endure an illness that has been mistakenly attributed to hypoglycemia.

Unfortunately, physicians often fail to recognize the symptoms of hypoglycemia. When actor Burt Reynolds made public his plight with hypoglycemia, most of us were astonished to learn that his condition went undiagnosed for many months, even with the best medical care. "I was sick for a whole year," Burt complained. "At the beginning, nobody could figure out what was wrong with me. I was so sick I honestly thought I'd die!"

If you have any of the symptoms of hypoglycemia that have not been attributed to a specific disorder, ask your doctor about testing you for low blood sugar. A five-hour glucose tolerance test, which is a series of blood tests performed at half-hour intervals after drinking a glucose solution, will uncover a blood sugar problem. An abnormally elevated blood sugar may mean diabetes, while an abnormal fall in blood sugar may point to functional or organic hypoglycemia.

Functional hypoglycemia is usually the result of pancreatic sensitivity caused by bad eating habits. *Organic hypoglycemia* may be the result of a pancreatic tumor or some other organic disease. Obviously, you must depend upon a physician for a correct diagnosis. Generally, the fasting blood sugar is consistently low in the case of organic hypoglycemia, especially in the morning before breakfast. In functional hypoglycemia, the blood sugar drops drastically a few hours after eating a refined carbohydrate.

Self-Treatment for Functional Hypoglycemia

Once it has been determined that hypoglycemia is the problem and that it is *functional* in nature rather than organic, the treatment is primarily up to you. The recommended dietary treatment may be used by anyone. In fact, the type of diet recommended for the treatment and prevention of hypoglycemia is the type of diet most of us should be on anyway. All of us should eat fresh, natural foods and avoid refined carbohydrates. It's perfectly all right to snack on natural foods between meals if you stay within your calorie requirement.

In the case of functional hypoglycemia, it's usually recommended that between-meal snacks consist of protein foods so that slower absorption and conversion of nutrients will maintain your blood sugar level without any drastic or sudden elevations. Remember, however, that if you eat protein snacks between meals and you are on a reducing diet, you must deduct the calorie value of the snacks from your calorie intake at mealtime. This won't be hard to do since a protein snack will reduce your appetite for a large meal.

Automatic Correction of Hypoglycemia

Luckily, your macro-nutrient diet will probably automatically eliminate symptoms of hypoglycemia. Marc F., an airline pilot who went on a macro-nutrient diet to reduce his body weight, reported that he experienced some unusual and unexpected benefits from his diet. "I was suffering from weak spells accompanied by sweating, trembling, and inability to concentrate," he said. "And I often got very sleepy during the day. All of this made flying very dangerous for me and my passengers. These problems disappeared, however, after only a couple of days on my new diet. I lost 36 pounds of fat, but I'm more pleased with the way I feel."

Marc was a victim of functional hypoglycemia and didn't know it. When he eliminated his coffee and doughnut snacks in following the macro-nutrient principles of dieting, he also eliminated his recurring hypoglycemia.

Many people who switch to a diet of fresh, natural foods report rejuvenation accompanied by increased energy and clearer thinking. This is often the result of correction of a blood sugar problem or a nutritional deficiency. When symptoms persist, it may be necessary to include a protein snack between meals.

High-Protein Snacks

Half a cup of yogurt (about 60 calories) mixed with a couple of teaspoons of miller's bran is a good fiber-rich, protein-rich snack for overweight persons. A little fresh fruit can be added for sweetening if desired. A celery stalk stuffed with cottage cheese or yogurt makes a good snack. Or you may simply eat yogurt or cottage cheese with fresh fruit.

A piece of baked chicken on a slice of whole-grain bread provides fiber along with protein. Toasted soybeans, raw sunflower seeds, bran cereal, corn pone with sesame seeds, a handful of homemade granola, natural peanut butter on whole-grain bread, and skim milk also provide energy-sustaining protein for between-meal snacks. Fresh fruit makes a good snack for most of us. But if you suffer from hypoglycemia, you should include some protein in your snacks. Cheese or peanut butter eaten with fresh fruit is a good fiber-rich protein snack. You must make sure, however, that the cheese is not of the processed variety and that the peanut butter has not been hydrogenated.

4. HOW TO KILL YOUR APPETITE
WITH ZERO-CALORIE FIBER

If you're on a low-calorie diet and you want to eat between meals to keep your stomach full, bran nibbling might be best for you. Unprocessed miller's bran provides bulk without calories and makes an ideal "stomach filler" for calorie-deficit eating. Since the phytates in bran can block absorption of minerals, large amounts of bran should not be eaten with meals. Between meals, however, when no other foods are eaten, pure bran can be eaten freely and safely.

Remember that you must absorb at least 1,200 nutrient-rich calories each day to stay healthy. So don't try to substitute bran for food at mealtime. A diet that's high in natural carbohydrate will supply all the fiber you need in your meals. This is one reason why you can eat generous amounts of natural carbohydrates without getting fat. Primitive Africans consume about 600 grams of natural carbohydrate and more than 3,000 calories a day without gaining weight. Take a lesson from the aborigines and include fiber-rich natural carbohydrates in every meal. It's all right to consume pure bran between meals. But at mealtime, *the foods you eat should supply the fiber you need.*

How to Use Bran to Prevent Constipation

Since bran is about 12 percent fiber, a good portion of the bran you consume will pass through your intestinal tract to form water-holding bulk in your colon. If there is adequate fiber in your diet, you won't suffer from constipation. If you *supplement* your diet with bran, your stools will be soft, bulky, moist, and easy to pass. (A gift from Heaven if you suffer from hemorrhoids!)

Bran provides more indigestible fiber than any other food product. As you learned earlier, the cellulose supplied by raw fruits and vegetables can be broken down to some extent by intestinal bacteria, so that only a small amount of fiber reaches the colon. A little extra bran in your diet will do wonders for your bowels *and* your weight.

How Much Bran Is Enough?

When bran is used as a supplement, it's generally recommended that adults consume about two teaspoons three times a day. This is often sprinkled over foods or taken with water just before eating. In order to avoid the mineral-blocking effect of the phytates in bran, however, it might be best to take bran *between* means when it is used in large amounts in a reducing diet. This will allow a greater intake of bran without nutritional interference. You may, in fact, use bran to replace calorie-rich snacks.

When you first begin using bran as a snack, you might experience an increase in intestinal gas. This usually disappears after six weeks or so. You may then increase your intake of bran at the rate of an extra teaspoon a day—as long as your stools are moist, firm, and regular. When your stools begin to get too loose or too frequent, you should cut back on your intake of bran.

Actually, bran is not an intestinal irritant. Too much bran, however, might adversely affect the water content of the colon by disturbing its osmotic balance. So begin with only a couple of teaspoons of bran and slowly increase the amount if there are no adverse effects.

Simple Bran Snacks

One of the best ways to snack on bran is to moisten it with skim milk so that it can be eaten as a mush. If you like, you can mix bran with wheat germ to make a larger, tastier snack. Plain miller's bran that has been moistened does not have a bad taste. In fact, bran actually has a pleasant wheaty taste—and it is chewy and easy to eat.

As you become more accustomed to the taste and the effect of bran, you can increase the proportion of bran to wheat germ. I personally like the taste of plain, moistened miller's bran, and I find it pleasant to chew.

If you do not like the taste of bran, you can mix it with yogurt or your favorite bran cereal.

Drink a glass of water immediately following a bran snack so that the bran can absorb enough moisture to multiply its bulk. Your stomach will then feel full and you won't be hungry.

When you reach your weight goal and you increase your calorie intake on a maintenance diet, you should substitute fresh fruit or some other wholesome, natural food for bran snacks. Or you may simply discontinue snacks and eat a little more food at mealtime. Just make sure that the foods you eat supply the fiber and the nutrients you need to maintain a healthy body weight.

SUMMARY

1. *Nibbling on high-fiber foods between meals will help cut your calorie intake by reducing your appetite at mealtime.*

2. *The method of nibbling you choose should depend upon the type of snacks you prefer, the type of diet you're on, and other factors.*
3. *Your daily food intake, supplying the number of calories you need, can be divided into three meals and three snacks to allow you to eat five or six times a day.*
4. *Persons who nibble compulsively or habitually should snack on raw vegetables.*
5. *Fiber-rich protein snacks such as stuffed celery or a handful of toasted soybeans may be best for victims of hypoglycemia.*
6. *Remember that between-meal snacks must not increase your calorie intake above what you need to reduce your body weight or to maintain your ideal weight.*
7. *Persons on a low-calorie reducing diet may be able to control their hunger by snacking on zero-calorie miller's bran between meals.*
8. *A tablespoon of miller's bran mixed with a little wheat germ and moistened with skim milk makes a filling low-calorie snack.*
9. *Bran intake may be increased at the rate of one teaspoon a day if no ill effects result.*
10. *Bran snacks should be replaced by fruits and other low-calorie foods when a reducing diet is replaced by a maintenance diet.*

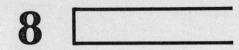

8

Fun and Purpose
in Eating Macro-Nutrient Foods
Away from Home

There's an old saying that "Some people eat to live, while others live to eat." Judging from the number of overweight people in America, most of us live to eat. Rather than eating to improve our health and nourish our bodies, we eat for taste and for pleasure. Eating out has become a form of recreation. We entertain friends by taking them to the nicest and most exclusive restaurant in town. When we go out in the evening, we try a new restaurant or a new type of food. Instead of exercising, we eat. And when we eat in restaurants more often than we eat at home, it's practically impossible to control or measure our intake of nutrients and calories.

RESTAURANT FOODS ARE OFTEN LOW IN NUTRIENTS

Food prepared in restaurants is often high in calories and deficient in vitamins. Storage, washing, cooking, heating, and delayed serving of foods results in loss of vitamins that are sensitive to light, heat, air, and water. But calories are unaffected. In fact, improper preparation of foods *reduces* their nutritional value while *increasing* their calorie value. An overcooked vegetable, for example, especially when boiled in water, may lose most of its water-soluble vitamins and minerals. If the vegetable has been cooked to a mush, it will supply more calories than a raw or slightly cooked vegetable. Furthermore, if fat or oil is added as a seasoning, the calorie content of the vegetable is greatly increased. Obviously, it would be difficult to operate your reducing power pedal for quick weight loss if you eat in restaurants often.

Except in a few health-oriented restaurants, the tendency is to cook foods in fat, especially in fast-food establishments. Sauces, oils, seasoning, and other ingredients added to casseroles and fancy dishes add calories on top of calories. *The only way you can be assured of getting maximum nutrients with minimum calories is to prepare your foods at home.* Steaming a little cabbage or lightly boiling a few green beans for *immediate* serving, for example, will assure a dependable source of low-calorie nutrients. Try to prepare fresh foods at home *each day,* especially if you are overweight.

When you do eat in restaurants, you should look for nutritious foods that are low in calories. This usually means selecting simple, basic foods that have been prepared without grease or oil. And it means eliminating visible fat, such as meat fat, butter, and salad dressing. You must also eliminate foods that are rich in *hidden* fat, such as pastries, white bread, and pies. Unfortunately, it's often difficult to tell whether restaurant-cooked vegetables contain fat or not. They may even contain sugar! Regardless, vegetables cooked in restaurants are likely to be overcooked and drained of nutrients. You cannot depend upon someone else's cooked vegetables to meet the needs of your reducing diet. So what *can* you eat when you dine out?

SELECTING SUITABLE MACRO-NUTRIENT FOODS
WHEN DINING OUT

It's always best to eat at home whenever possible. When you do plan to eat out, it might be a good idea to reduce your appetite by eating something at home *before* you go out. You may then nibble on a raw salad or a fruit dish just to be good company for your companion.

For a complete meal, order a raw salad, but skip the salad dressing. A little salt or lemon juice is all the dressing you need. You don't need croutons, either, especially if you have a couple of whole-grain crackers. Meat dishes should be lean, unfried, and without gravy. Roast beef or broiled fish, for example, would be a good choice. Baked chicken would be fine if you peel off the skin. Remember that the most expensive meats are usually the fattiest. Prime rib and choice steaks, for example, are tender because they are high in fat. So they are more expensive.

Pick one or two of the plainest vegetables on the menu, such as cabbage, string beans, or greens. Stay away from casseroles and other dishes that contain a variety of ingredients. Since restaurant vegetables often contain oil or sugar, try to get by with one vegetable. You can't go wrong with a baked potato. If you eat a whole baked potato and a raw salad with roast beef or broiled fish, you won't need anything else to eat. Unsweetened tea, skim milk, water, or vegetable juice makes a good beverage for a low-calorie meal.

Unfortunately, few restaurants serve skim milk. If you must have coffee with cream, take along a little skim milk powder to replace the cream. Non-dairy creamers are usually made with saturated fat, such as coconut oil. This means that they contain harmful fat as well as extra calories.

Cut Calories in Half by Eliminating Visible Fat

Simply eliminating the fat you can *see* in your meal will greatly reduce your calorie intake. Fat contains nine calories per gram while protein and carbohydrate each contain only four calories per gram. Of course, carbohydrates must be *natural*. Refined carbohydrates such as sugar, white bread, spaghetti, pastries, and other processed foods are absorbed so easily and so rapidly that they stimulate storage of body fat by triggering production of insulin. Thus, the four calories supplied by one gram of a fruit, a vegetable, or a whole-grain product may not be as fattening as the four calories supplied by one gram of sugar or white flour.

After making sure that you eat natural carbohydrates instead of refined, fiber-deficient carbohydrates, the next most important step to be taken is to reduce your intake of fat—as recommended in *Dietary Goals.* When refined carbohydrates have been eliminated from your diet and fats have been reduced to a minimum, your fat-burner throttle will begin to function effectively. Fat will begin to disappear as if by magic.

Lose Fat Permanently with Natural Carbohydrates

At this point, you're probably asking, "If fat is more fattening than carbohydrate, then why do some people lose weight on a high-fat, low-carbohydrate diet? One reason, of course, is that when you eliminate a major energy nutrient such as carbohydrate you automatically reduce your intake of calories. Simply eliminating *refined* carbohydrates will greatly reduce the calorie intake of most Americans. Since foods rich in fat have great satiety value, you simply do not eat as much when you eat a lot of fat. But a high-fat diet is not a healthful diet. If your diet is deficient in natural carbohydrate, you'll lose more muscle protein and body water than fat. Even if you do lose some body fat on a high-fat diet, a large intake of fat can contribute to the development of cancer, hardened arteries, and other diseases.

Remember what I told you in earlier chapters of this book: *Natural carbohydrates, which are rich in fiber and water, are not as fattening as refined carbohydrates and fat-rich foods.* This is one reason why the new U.S. Dietary Goals recommend that such a high percentage of your energy should be supplied by natural carbohydrates. Avoid refined and fatty foods, especially when you eat out. Forget about the popular low-carbohydrate diets that allow a large intake of fat. Concentrate on natural, low-fat foods. Eliminate visible fat whenever possible.

How to Manipulate the Fat in Your Meals

In Chapter 4, I gave you an example of how you can reduce the calorie content of a steakhouse meal simply by eliminating fat. A typical meal consisting of an eight-ounce rib steak, a baked potato with butter and sour cream, a mixed green salad with French dressing, hot rolls with butter, and coffee with cream and sugar, for example, supplies about 1,660 calories! If you substitute four ounces of ground round steak or some broiled fish for the rib steak, two slices of whole-wheat bread for the dinner rolls, and eliminate the butter, the sour cream, the French dressing, and the cream and sugar, you can add one-half cup each of two vegetables to your meal and still not take in more than 650 calories! And by adding two vegetable dishes, you are adding valuable fiber. The whole-wheat bread also supplies fiber.

Obviously, the foods you choose when you eat out can make the difference between being fat or being lean. If you eat out a lot, choose your foods carefully. Don't hesitate to ask for the foods you want or to reject the foods you don't want.

A Sample Low-Fat Meal

A meal consisting of a mixed green salad, a cup of skim milk, one-half cup of string beans, one baked potato, four ounces of broiled fish, and one slice of whole wheat bread supplies about 465 calories. You can eat all the green salad you want as long as you don't use salad dressing.

Unfortunately, it's practically impossible to get real whole-grain bread in a restaurant. So it might be best to skip the bread. It may also be difficult to get skim milk. A cup of whole milk supplies *twice* as many calories as a cup of skim milk. When skim milk isn't available, it would be better to drink water with your meal and then have a glass of skim milk and a slice of whole-grain bread as a between-meal snack at home. Your meal would then supply only 315 calories, and the between-meal snack 150 calories.

Thus, with a little planning and a little knowledge, you can select a few appropriate foods when you eat in a restaurant and then balance your food intake with between-meal snacks (see Chapter 7).

TIPS FROM CELEBRITIES ON EATING OUT

Health-conscious celebrities who travel a great deal can offer us some valuable tips on eating out.* Actor *Ed Asner,* for example, avoids fast-food establishments where foods are usually fried. "When I eat out," he says, "I never eat in restaurants where the foods are steeped in grease."

John Beradino of TV's "General Hospital" doesn't risk ordering new or unfamiliar foods. "I really don't experiment with foods," he states emphatically. "Even when I go to an Italian restaurant,

Peter Lupus' Celebrity Body Book, by Peter Lupus and Samuel Homola, Parker Publishing Company, West Nyack, New York, 1980.

I'll probably have shrimp scampi with garlic; that's one of my favorites. When I find something I like, I stick with it."

Movie star *Peter Lawford* also avoids experimenting with foods when he eats out. "When I eat out," he explained, "I usually order something I'm familiar with, such as scrambled eggs. I don't like rich foods, such as sauces and so on."

TV comedian *Ted Knight* checks the cook as well as the kitchen when he eats out! "I'm very selective when I eat out, but it's never as good as when I eat at home," he observed. "So I always take double doses of supplemental vitamins with me. I avoid sauces and things of that nature, and I make certain that the salads are cleansed properly. I even check the kitchen. I want to know who the cooks are and how they prepare the food before I eat it. I try to avoid restaurants as much as I can. I don't eat fried stuff at all. I'll seek out vegetables on my plate more than I will the main course and then cut my supply in half."

Comedian *Paul Lynde* has found that restaurant meals are usually fattening. "When I'm on the road," he says, "I try to limit my diet to a broiled piece of meat or seafood and a big salad. But I'm never hungry before giving a performance. So I usually eat *after* a performance. Unfortunately, it's usually so late when I get out of the theater that there aren't any good restaurants open. If someone stays open for you and they know you're coming, they want you to eat the specialty of the house, which is usually fattening."

Take Your Own Lunch

When Broadway singer and comedienne Carol Channing eats away from home, she usually takes along her own lunch in a bag and her drinking water in a thermos. She does this to make sure that her meal consists of fresh, natural food and pure water that is free of additives.

When you are on a strict low-calorie diet, you, too, can carry your own lunch wherever you go, whether you're going to work or to a restaurant with a friend. Or you may carry *part* of your lunch. If you go to a restaurant, for example, you can order the meat dish or the salad or whatever you want and then balance your meal with fresh fruit, whole-grain bread, and other foods you've brought along to complete your meal. If you feel embarrassed doing this, think of Ted Knight and Carol Channing, both of whom refuse to sacrifice their health by being intimidated into eating bad foods in public places.

Desserts are also a problem in restaurants. If raw fruit or melon isn't available and you must have something sweet, take along a few raisins or some fresh or dried fruit. A baked sweet potato makes a satisfying fiber-rich dessert. It would be better to do without dessert than to eat the sugary, fatty, or synthetic desserts served in most restaurants. Picture yourself as a prisoner in a cocoon of fat and you won't have any trouble saying "no" to artificial desserts.

How Eunice P. Lost 35 Pounds Eating Out

Eunice P. spent most of her time traveling as a cosmetic representative. Since she was about 40 pounds overweight, it was obvious that she wasn't eating properly. "I've just about given up," she admitted. "When I'm eating out, I really do not know what to eat."

I told Eunice about macro-nutrient foods, that is, about fresh, natural foods prepared without fat. Once she got the idea, she was able to select a few basic foods in restaurants and then keep her diet balanced with lunches and snacks consisting of fruit, cheese, and other healthful foods. Although Eunice never bothered to keep a record of her calorie intake, she managed to lose 35 pounds in two months. How did she do it?

Conscientious elimination of sugar, fat, and refined carbohydrates from her diet was the primary reason for Eunice's dieting success. The satiety value of fiber-rich natural carbohydrates made it much easier for her to control her appetite. "I now take along fresh fruits, vegetables, and whole-grain bread when I travel," she explained, "and I frequently shop in a grocery store for my meals. I really like my new way of eating. Even if I no longer had a weight problem, I would never revert to dependence upon restaurants for all my meals."

After you have completed this chapter, you, too, will be able to stay on your diet when you travel or eat away from home. You'll develop new ways of eating that will become a part of your way of life. Best of all, you'll discover taste treats that will make eating exciting and more pleasurable.

VARIETY IN YOUR LUNCH BOX

There are many nutritious low-calorie foods that you can pack in a box or a bag for lunch on the job or while traveling. You can choose from such foods as poultry, boiled eggs, baked potatoes, cottage cheese, whole-grain bread, yogurt, fresh fruit, raw vegetables, canned juices, raw seeds and nuts, dried fruit, and so on. Just make sure that the foods are fresh and natural and not prepared with grease or oil. And no mayonnaise! Try to include something from each of the basic four food groups. Foods from the *milk group* (such as cottage cheese), the *vegetable-fruit group* (such as tomatoes and apples), the *meat group* (such as baked chicken), and the *bread-cereal group* (such as whole wheat bread), for example, will assure a balanced diet.

If you cook your vegetables without grease, oil, or fat, you can pack cooked vegetables in small plastic containers and have them for lunch. A cold, cooked vegetable is delicious if it is not laced with grease. Corn pone baked in an oven (Chapter 6) is not greasy and is also delicious cold.

Avoid Lunch Meats

When you pack meat sandwiches in your lunch box, use fresh meat, such as sliced roast beef, baked chicken, or ground round steak. Make sure that the meat is well cooked. Try not to keep meat in an unrefrigerated lunch box longer than four hours before eating. You should always keep your lunch box in a cool place.

Lunch meats that have been preserved with additives won't readily spoil. But some preservatives, such as sodium nitrite, might be harmful to your body. Lunch meats might also contain sugar, salt, monosodium glutamate, and other undesirable ingredients. Salt and monosodium glutamate can trigger migraine headache in some people. "The Chinese restaurant syndrome," or flushing and palpitation of the heart, has been traced to excessive use of monosodium glutamate as a seasoning. Sodium nitrite or nitrate preservatives tend to cause a drop in blood pressure and pulse rate along with flushing and headache. Such symptoms can affect job performance as well as create a safety hazard. So it might be a good idea to avoid consumption of lunch meats whenever possible.

Be Careful Not to Overeat

Overeating can affect your job performance adversely. When your stomach is too full, it's more difficult to concentrate and move around. If you want to feel well, work efficiently, and lose weight, put fresh natural foods in your lunch box—and don't overeat! A boiled egg, a baked potato, a piece of fresh fruit, and a slice of Swiss cheese between two slices of whole-grain bread is not a fancy lunch, but it can be filling, satisfying, and healthful, with only 415 calories. If you include a glass of water with your lunch, you may even have difficulty finishing your meal.

Snacking on the Job

A between-meal snack on the job will take the edge off your appetite so that you don't eat so much at mealtime. A piece of fresh fruit will be best for most of us. If you eat anything other than fresh fruit or raw vegetables, make sure that your snacks fall within your calorie requirement.

Turn back to Chapter 7 and review the various methods of snacking. Select the method that best suits your needs. If you suffer from hypoglycemia, for example, you'll need a protein snack such as cottage cheese or baked chicken. If you are on an extremely low-calorie diet, you may have to snack on milk-moistened bran to kill your hunger by filling your stomach. Bran mixed with a small amount of yogurt makes a chewy, filling snack.

Try a Grocery Store When Traveling

When you are traveling in your car, it might be a good idea to shop in a grocery store for some of your meals. You can buy skim milk, low-fat cottage cheese or yogurt, fresh fruit, your favorite cheese, whole-grain bread, juice, and raw vegetables such as celery, carrots, tomatoes, and lettuce. You can eat such foods in your car or in a park area along the highway.

Cheese and whole-grain bread with fresh fruit will meet your nutritional requirements very well. You don't need to eat meat if you include a dairy product such as cheese. A little dried fruit can supply the iron you would normally get from meat.

Eating raw foods for a few days while traveling is a great way to clean your intestines. It would even be all right to "fast" for a couple of days on fresh fruits and juices. If you choose to go on a total fast for a day or two, you should at least drink vegetable juice. In addition to being low in calories, vegetable juice helps neutralize the acids that accumulate in your system when you fast. Fruit juices also have an alkaline effect in your body, but it would be better to eat the whole fruit rather than squeeze it for juice. The fiber in raw fruits will reduce calorie intake as well as provide healthful bulk for your intestine.

Remember that it's never a good idea to eliminate any of the basic foods for more than a day or two. You must have nutrients from each of the basic food groups each day for the best of health.

SUPPLEMENT QUESTIONABLE DIETS WITH VITAMINS

In an earlier chapter, I suggested that diets that supply less than 2,000 calories a day, even when balanced with natural foods, should be supplemented with vitamins. In addition to a possible dietary deficiency, vitamins may also be lost in the preparation of food. Water-soluble vitamins, for example, can be easily lost to heat, light, air, water, and other factors. When calorie intake is reduced to a level where vitamin intake may be barely adequate, you must supplement your diet to make up for possible losses as well as for a dietary deficiency.

Minerals are not easily destroyed, but some are water soluble. So it might be a good idea to include minerals in a good multiple vitamin and mineral formula when supplementing a low-calorie reducing diet.

How to Supplement Your Diet with Water-Soluble Vitamins

It's especially important to supplement your diet with the water-soluble vitamins when you are reducing your body weight. Vitamin B complex and Vitamin C, for example, must be supplied daily since they cannot be stored and can be flushed from your body by water. An increased elimination of water by your kidneys as a result of burning body fat can flush vitamins *and* minerals from your body.

Remember that a carbohydrate-deficient diet results in excessive loss of body water and water-soluble nutrients without much loss of body fat. Be sure to keep your diet balanced so that at least

48 percent of your energy intake comes from natural carbohydrate.

When you take B vitamins, you should take all of them in the form of "B complex." The B vitamins work together, and taking only one B vitamin may create a deficiency in other B vitamins. Any moderately potent B complex formula will do fine. Your body will simply excrete unused B vitamins, turning your urine a bright yellow.

Your body will also excrete unused Vitamin C. According to the Food and Nutrition Board of the National Research Council, the average healthy adult needs only about 60 milligrams of Vitamin C daily. If you smoke cigarettes, however, or if you are ill or under stress, you may need considerably more Vitamin C than usual to prevent a deficiency. When you are on a reducing diet, you may need extra Vitamin C to replace that lost in the elimination of water from your body.

How to Take Larger Doses of Vitamins Safely

If you want to take vitamins in large doses without professional supervision, you can do so safely if you stay within a reasonable range. (See Table 8-1.) Here's a guide that anyone can follow—from Recommended Dietary Allowances (RDA) to larger doses for nutritional insurance. (For additional information on vitamins and minerals, see *Recommended Dietary Allowances*, 9th Edition, published by the National Academy of Sciences, 2101 Constitution Avenue, N.W., Washington, D.C. 20418, 1980.)

RDA	Larger Dose
Vitamin A, 5,000 units	10,000 units
Folic Acid, 400 micrograms	400 micrograms
Niacinamide, 19 milligrams	50 milligrams
Riboflavin, 1.7 milligrams	10 milligrams
Thiamine, 1.5 milligrams	10 milligrams
Pyridoxine (B_6), 2.2 milligrams	10 milligrams
Vitamin B_{12}, 3 micrograms	10 micrograms
Vitamin C (ascorbic acid), 60 milligrams	500 milligrams
Vitamin D, 400 units	400 units
Vitamin E (mixed), 12 units	200 units

Table 8-1

Note: I usually refer to the Recommended Dietary Allowances (RDAs) as the recommended *Daily* Allowances, since dietary allowances are figured on a daily basis. The Recommended Dietary

Allowances should not be confused with the U.S. Recommended Dietary Allowances (U.S. RDAs). The RDAs represent the amounts of nutrients recommended by the Food and Nutrition Board of the National Research Council for maintaining good health in healthy persons. The U.S. RDAs (or MDRs) are the amounts of protein, vitamins, and minerals established by the Food and Drug Administration as standards for nutrition labeling. The MDRs, or Minimum Daily Requirements, are believed to be adequate to prevent symptoms of a deficiency but may be less than the Recommended Dietary Allowances.

The suggested larger doses of the water-soluble vitamins (B and C) are, of course, flexible. Water-soluble vitamins can be taken in fairly large doses safely. But the larger the dose the more expensive the vitamin and, except in special cases, larger doses may not be necessary. Extremely large doses of any vitamin might create problems. Persons having trouble with gouty arthritis or kidney stones, for example, should be cautious about taking more than a few thousand milligrams of Vitamin C daily. (More than 4,000 milligrams of Vitamin C daily might contribute to the formation of oxalic acid stones.) According to the National Academy of Sciences, Vitamin B6 dependency has been induced in normal human adults by feeding them 200 milligrams of Vitamin B6 daily for 33 days while they were ingesting a normal diet. The same may hold true for other vitamins. Taking large doses of Vitamin C for a long period of time can result in a temporary rebound effect when the dosage is discontinued. So if you're the average healthy person taking vitamins for nutritional insurance, select a potency somewhere between the RDA and the larger dose I've listed.

Remember that the fat-soluble vitamins (A,D,E, and K) can be stored in your body. It's well known that overdoses of Vitamins A and D can be toxic. It might be best, therefore, not to take more than 10,000 units of Vitamin A daily if the foods in your diet also supply Vitamin A. A healthy adult's requirement for Vitamin D can be met by exposure to sunlight. Most of us, however, should make sure that our diet supplies us with at least 400 units of Vitamin D daily. (More than 2,000 units of Vitamin D daily could result in retention of too much calcium.) Egg yolk, fish, liver, butter, sunflower seeds, and fortified milk are among the few dietary sources of Vitamin D. No toxic effects have yet been observed in persons taking large doses of Vitamin E—but be cautious.

You should not be taking larger and larger doses of any vitamin without a good reason. Keep your diet balanced to *prevent* a deficiency. Take only moderate doses of vitamins for added protection. Then, when you need larger doses of vitamins for medical reasons, you should seek professional guidance.

PREVENTING CALCIUM AND IRON DEFICIENCIES

Calcium and iron are commonly deficient in American diets. Women who are pregnant or who menstruate heavily need extra iron, and there may be a need for additional calcium after menopause. Anyone on a low-calorie diet is likely to be deficient in iron.

Calcium Must Be Supplied Daily

The Recommended Daily Allowance for calcium ranges from 800 to 1,200 milligrams a day, depending upon age, sex, and other factors. A pregnant or lactating woman, for example, needs 1,200 milligrams of calcium daily. It has been estimated that *about 700 milligrams of calcium enter and leave the bones of the average adult each day*. Since your bones are constantly being formed and resorbed, you must supply your body with calcium *daily* to keep your bones strong. Your body *loses* about 320 milligrams of calcium daily. Only about 40 percent of the calcium you consume is absorbed. This means that your foods should supply about 800 milligrams of calcium each day to meet normal needs. This is one reason why your reducing diet should always include calcium-rich dairy products.

If your diet supplies adequate calcium, your body will absorb what it needs and eliminate the rest. But remember that it's important to keep your diet *balanced*. Too much meat in your diet, for example, supplying an excessive amount of phosphorus, will force your body to eliminate an excessive amount of calcium. And when there is not adequate Vitamin D in your diet, your body cannot utilize calcium in rebuilding bones.

A macro-nutrient diet, if followed as instructed, will protect you from deficiencies while your body weight is being reduced.

Too Much Iron Can Be Toxic

The diet of the average man or woman should supply from 10 to 18 milligrams of iron daily—about 10 milligrams for men and 18 milligrams for women of child-bearing age. Your body does not actually use this much iron. You need only one or two milligrams of iron daily to make up for losses and to maintain your reserves if you are healthy. But since you absorb only about 10 percent of the iron in your diet, you must consume 18 milligrams of iron to supply your body with 1.8 milligrams of usable iron.

The ordinary diet does not supply more than 18 milligrams of iron. An adult woman who does not *exceed* her recommended calorie requirement will consume only nine to 12 milligrams of iron daily. Obviously, women of child-bearing age, persons suffering from anemia, and other people who need more iron than the ordinary diet supplies must take an iron supplement to maintain iron reserves. Too much supplemental iron can be toxic, however, and not all types of anemia can be corrected by taking iron. If you are anemic, you should be treated by a physician who can prescribe iron and other measures according to your needs.

Getting Your Iron from Foods

Unless you are on an unbalanced or iron-deficient diet (less than 2,000 calories) and you are anemic, or unless you are pregnant or menstruating, you may not need an iron supplement. If blood tests show that your red cells are carrying a full quota of iron and you're not losing blood, you should be cautious with iron supplements. Excess iron can accumulate in your body and cause symptoms of iron poisoning.

Try to get the iron you need from the foods you eat and then supplement your diet only when necessary to prevent or correct a deficiency. Your body will absorb only the amount of iron it needs from natural foods. Unnecessary use of iron supplements, however, may force absorption of more iron than your body can use.

Liver and other meats are good sources of iron. *Eating a piece of citrus fruit with your meat sandwich will increase absorption of iron.* This is another good reason why you should keep your diet balanced, especially when you are on a low-calorie diet. But remember: When you are on a reducing diet and your calorie intake falls below 2,000 calories, iron should be included in your multiple vitamin and mineral supplement. If you are a woman and you menstruate, you may need additional iron even if you eat normally.

Note: Taking Vitamin E with iron in supplement form might interfere with absorption of iron. Don't mix Vitamin E pills with iron pills if you are being treated for anemia. Iron and Vitamin E supplied by natural foods, however, are absorbed normally.

EVERYONE'S NEEDS ARE DIFFERENT

According to the National Academy of Sciences, the Recommended Daily Allowances for vitamins and minerals are approximate estimates "Designed for the maintenance of good nutrition of practically all healthy people in the U.S.A." Unfortunately, most people are not truly healthy, and everyone's needs are not exactly the same. Furthermore, some *healthy* persons need more of some nutrients than others. Although the Recommended Daily Allowances are estimated to *exceed* the requirements of most individuals, thereby ensuring that the needs of nearly all are met, many people maintain that they feel better taking extra vitamins. If you feel that your needs exceed the Recommended Daily Allowances, you can use supplements in order to meet these needs without increasing your calorie intake. Of course, when you are on a low-calorie reducing diet, you would certainly be deficient in some of the essential vitamins and minerals if you did not supplement your diet with *at least* the Recommended Daily Allowances.

Extra Vitamins for Special Reasons

When you are ill, your doctor may prescribe large doses of selected vitamins and minerals—usually vitamins—for therapeutic purposes. Vitamins A and C, for example, may be prescribed in combating infection. Vitamin C is often used to strengthen weak blood vessels and tissue collagen. The B vitamins have been used in the treatment of skin and nervous disorders. Vitamin E is believed to be of value in preventing blood clots and improving circulation. Calcium, Vitamin D, and magnesium are commonly employed to strengthen soft bones. Zinc has been found useful in speeding healing following injury or surgery. Women who take birth control pills may need additional Vitamin B₆. Alcoholics need big doses of B vitamins. Smokers need extra Vitamin C, and so on.

Obviously, many people can benefit from large doses of vitamins and minerals in special cases. Megadoses of any nutrient must be monitored as a drug, by a physician, so don't arbitrarily dose yourself with extremely large amounts of any nutrient. Just try to make sure that you reasonably exceed your Recommended Daily Allowances—whether you eat at home or carry your lunch.

SUMMARY

1. *Your first reason for eating should be to nourish your body rather than to pamper your taste.*
2. *Whenever you have a choice, it's always best to prepare your meals at home rather than eat out.*
3. *When you do eat out, select simple, basic foods such as roast beef, baked potato, and green salad.*
4. *You cannot depend upon restaurant-cooked vegetables for your vitamins, so always try to prepare your vegetables at home.*
5. *If you must eat out frequently, eat less by avoiding forbidden foods and then eat a between-meal snack to supply needed nutrients.*
6. *The calorie content of restaurant meals can be greatly reduced simply by eliminating visible fat.*
7. *When you work and you are consistently unable to eat at home, you should learn how to pack a healthful lunch.*
8. *When you are traveling in your car, you can pick up a healthful meal in almost any grocery store.*
9. *Low-calorie diets should always be supplemented with the Recommended Daily Allowance of vitamins and minerals, especially when you eat out.*
10. *Persons who need therapeutic doses of vitamins and minerals to treat an illness or to correct a deficiency should seek the guidance of a nutritionally oriented physician.*

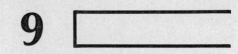

9

The Lifetime
Health-and-Body Benefits
of Macro-Nutrient Foods

When the U.S. Department of Agriculture published *Human Nutrition* in 1971, the report stated that "Most all of the health problems underlying the leading causes of death in the United States could be modified by improvements in diet." Then, in 1977, the U.S. Senate Select Committee on Nutrition and Human Needs stated in *Dietary Goals for the United States* that "In all, six of the ten leading causes of death in the United States have been linked to our diet."

Obviously, what you eat can have a great deal to do with your health and your longevity. A poorly balanced diet that does not supply all the essential nutrients, or a diet that supplies an excessive amount of sugar, salt, fat, or artificial additives, can ruin your health and your body—whether you are overweight or not.

A REDUCING DIET THAT BUILDS GOOD HEALTH!

As you already know, the first step to be taken in eating to protect your health is eating fresh, natural foods in a balanced diet each day. Then, to guard against a buildup of body fat, you must exert reasonable control over the *amount* of food you eat. You must also adopt a diet plan that can be followed every day of your life without a hassle.

Wouldn't it be wonderful to have a diet plan that would improve your health and prolong your life while reducing excess body fat? Well, you have such a plan in this book. Supplying fiber as well as essential nutrients, my macro-nutrient diet will serve you for the rest of your life, and it will keep you healthy as well as lean. Following the general rules outlined in this book will help you *prevent* some of the leading causes of death!

Here's how the Bureau of the Census lists the 10 leading causes of death.

1. Diseases of the heart
2. Malignant neoplasms
3. Vascular lesions affecting the central nervous system
4. Accidents
5. Influenza and pneumonia
6. Certain diseases of early infancy
7. Diabetes mellitus
8. General arteriosclerosis
9. Other bronchopulmonic diseases
10. Cirrhosis of the liver

There are, of course, many factors that play a part in the development of disease, such as stress, heredity, smoking cigarettes, drinking alcohol, lack of exercise, and so on. But diet plays a major role in the development of all but four of the listed 10 leading causes of death. Although your macro-nutrient diet will essentially eliminate diet's role in contributing to the development of disease, there are some special dietary precautions that should be observed if you want maximum protection against disease.

How Eating Can Save Your Life

The importance of diet in controlling your body weight and protecting your health can probably best be appreciated by comparing the physical condition of someone who eats properly with someone who does not. Take the case of Andrew T., for example. He was a busy 60-year-old overweight architect whose hobby was cooking and eating. A routine examination in my office revealed that he was about 50 pounds overweight with abnormally elevated blood levels of cholesterol, glucose, and triglycerides. His blood pressure was 210 over 100 and his pulse rate a rapid 90 beats per minute, indicating a poor physical condition and an overworked heart.

Andrew was advised that if he didn't change his eating habits and do something about his weight, he might have a heart attack. "Just as soon as I get back from my tour of Europe, I'll do something about my diet," Andrew promised, punctuating his remark with cigar smoke.

When Andrew returned after spending a month in Europe, he was fatter than ever. A year later, I read his obituary in the local newspaper. Dead at 61!

Edward D. Chose to Live

Edward D. was also in poor physical condition when I first saw him in my office. A borderline diabetic, he feared the possibility of a need for insulin injections. A high level of blood sugar and blood fat threatened every artery in his body. I told Edward that if he would get rid of his excess body fat, chances are he would automatically reduce his blood sugar and blood fat. I didn't have to repeat this advice twice. Edward asked for a copy of the basic rules I've outlined in Chapter 1 of this book. Three months later, he had reduced his body weight by 38 pounds. After six months, he had shed a total of 52 pounds and was maintaining his ideal body weight. "My family physician now says that my blood sugar and blood fat are normal," Edward reported, expressing a new enthusiasm for life. "I really appreciate everything your diet has done for me."

I couldn't help but think of Andrew while listening to Edward. Andrew had died in the prime of his life, his heart and his muscles laboring against blood fat and body fat up to the last minute of his life. Edward, on the other hand, had transformed himself into a lean, healthy, and energetic person with a promise of unlimited longevity.

What about you? If you're fat and your health and your longevity are being threatened by diabetes, clogged arteries, or some other disease associated with obesity or a bad diet, you shouldn't have any trouble at all making a decision to change your eating habits. Eating properly is just as easy as eating improperly.

So there is no real sacrifice involved. All you have to do is make a few simple changes in your eating habits, so that you may live instead of die. It's up to you.

Check Your Blood Fat and Record Your Pulse Rate

Have your doctor check your blood sugar, cholesterol, and triglycerides. Ask for a copy of the results. Record your pulse rate. Your fasting blood sugar may range from 65 to 112 milligrams percent (per 100 milliliters of blood). Your cholesterol should be less than 200 milligrams percent, never above 300. Triglycerides should be lower than cholesterol, from 40 to 165 milligrams percent. When sugar, cholesterol, and triglycerides are above the high normals listed on lab reports, you're headed for trouble if changes aren't made.

The lower your pulse rate the less strain there is on your heart. Generally, when excess body fat is reduced, blood sugar, cholesterol, and triglycerides will also be reduced. These changes will usually be reflected in a lower pulse rate.

A normal pulse rate is about 72 beats per minute. If your resting pulse rate is above 80, you're probably in poor physical condition. *If your resting pulse rate is over 92, your chances of dying young are four times greater than if you had a resting pulse rate lower than 67.*

Note: Regular exercise will reduce blood levels of sugar, fat, and cholesterol as well as lower your pulse rate. So be sure to combine exercise with diet whenever possible. Exercise also burns calories, thus speeding loss of excess body fat.

Your pulse rate will be faster after smoking cigarettes, after drinking coffee or colas, and after eating. The best time to take your pulse is in the morning before eating or drinking and before facing the stress of a new day.

PREVENTING HEART AND BLOOD VESSEL DISEASE
WITH MACRO-NUTRIENT FOODS

Heart disease is America's No. 1 killer. Each year, 850,000 Americans die from heart and blood vessel disease. More than *half* of all deaths in America are attributed to cardiovascular disease!

Since the foods you eat have a great deal to do with the

development of cardiovascular disease, you obviously cannot afford to ignore your diet, even if you are not overweight. You can less afford to go on a high-protein, high-fat reducing diet that might contribute to the development of disease, so it's absolutely essential that you adopt a sensible diet plan that will assure protection for your heart and your blood vessels. This usually means a balanced diet of natural foods that will provide essential nutrients while preventing a buildup of cholesterol and fat in your blood.

Keeping Your Cholesterol Under Control

Although the cholesterol question is far from settled, there is little doubt that a high level of blood cholesterol, whatever its origin, is a factor in the development of cardiovascular disease. According to *Dietary Goals,* a plasma cholesterol level of 260 milligrams or higher per 100 milliliters of blood carries with it *five times* the risk of heart disease as compared to a level of 220 milligrams percent or lower. In societies where the level of plasma cholesterol is *under* 150 to 160 milligrams percent, there are virtually no deaths from heart disease!

Most doctors consider a plasma cholesterol level up to 250 to 300 milligrams percent to be normal. What is average or normal, however, is not necessarily optimal or healthful. Because the average American's diet is so bad, with such a high percentage of fat and refined carbohydrates, the average blood cholesterol is far too high. So even if your doctor tells you that your cholesterol level is "average," you should change your diet as necessary to get your cholesterol down to 180 milligrams percent or less.

Saturated Fat Builds Cholesterol

Cholesterol is not a fat, but it is associated with fats of animal origin. There is some evidence to indicate that the saturated fat in your diet might actually do more to raise your blood cholesterol than the cholesterol supplied by foods. In any event, lowering your intake of animal fat will reduce your intake of cholesterol *and* saturated fat. And since a high intake of any type of fat—saturated or unsaturated—might contribute to the development of cancer and other diseases, it's important to make sure that no more than 30 percent of your energy intake is supplied by fats and oils.

Balancing the macro-nutrients in your diet so that up to 58

percent of your energy intake comes from natural carbohydrate and at least 12 percent from protein will protect you against an excessive intake of saturated fat and cholesterol—provided, of course, that your foods are properly prepared (see Chapter 4). If you are healthy and your blood cholesterol is not already too high, you won't have to worry about the cholesterol and fat content of such wholesome foods as eggs and lean meat in a balanced diet.

Natural Carbohydrates Reduce Blood Cholesterol

The fiber supplied by complex (natural) carbohydrates in a macro-nutrient diet will help lower cholesterol and triglycerides (fat) in your blood, thus reducing the risk of heart disease. According to researchers quoted in *Dietary Goals*, population groups with the lowest incidence of coronary heart disease consume from 65 to 85 percent of their total energy in the form of carbohydrate derived from whole-grain cereals and potatoes. "High carbohydrate diets are quite appropriate for both normal individuals and for most of those with hyperlipidemia (high levels of fat in the blood), provided that the carbohydrate is largely derived from grains and tubers, that an energy excess is not consumed, and that adiposity does not result."

For lifelong protection against heart and blood vessel disease, you should pattern your eating habits after the new U.S. Dietary Goals (see Chapter 1). Forget about the high-protein, high-fat, low-carbohydrate diets that are now so popular. Keep your calorie intake down at a level recommended for your bone size and height. Depend upon *fresh fruits and vegetables and whole-grain products* to supply about 58 percent of your total calorie intake.

For additional protection against heart disease, be sure to eliminate sugar and white-flour products as much as possible. Cut away visible meat fat and do not cook with fat or oil. Employing such simple measures should not be too big a price to pay for lifelong protection against heart disease, hardened arteries, and stroke.

The Good Guys in Cholesterol

Although the total amount of cholesterol in your blood should not go above 180 milligrams percent, the *type* of cholesterol in your blood provides a good clue to your susceptibility to cardiovascular disease. There is a good cholesterol and a bad cholesterol, depending upon its carrier. Cholesterol and fat are transported in the blood by two types of lipoproteins—like cowboys riding horses.

Low-density lipoproteins (LDL), the "bad guys," transport cholesterol into the walls of arteries and other tissues, contributing to the development of disease.

High-density lipoproteins (HDL) are "good guys" who transport cholesterol to the liver where the cholesterol is converted to bile and excreted by the gall bladder. An increased amount of fiber in your diet, supplied by natural carbohydrates, helps lower blood cholesterol by stimulating excretion and elimination of bile. Some nutritionists believe that Vitamin C, lecithin, and other ingredients of natural foods increase the percentage of high-density lipoproteins in the blood.

Regular exercise is especially effective in stimulating the formation of high-density lipoproteins. In fact, researchers have reported that exercise is *more* effective than dietary measures in producing high-density lipoproteins. So even if your macronutrient diet lowers the total amount of cholesterol in your blood, a little regular exercise will help by changing bad cholesterol to good cholesterol. Exercise will also firm your muscles, burn excess body fat, and strengthen your heart, thus making you look better and feel better.

How to Strengthen Your Heart

For best results in strengthening your heart, work your way up to 20 to 30 minutes of exercise at least every other day. The exercise should be of sufficient intensity to keep your heart beating at 75 percent of its maximum capacity (at least 120 beats per minute). Or you may simply participate in forms of exercise that burn 300 or more calories in half an hour (10 calories a minute). Handball, jogging, and other endurance-type athletic activities burn about 10 calories a minute. Of course, the heavier you are the more calories you burn during physical activity. Most people can lose half a pound or more of body fat a week simply by spending 20 minutes a day in recreational exercise.

HOW TO FIGHT CANCER WITH A MACRO-NUTRIENT DIET

Cancer is the second most common cause of death in America. There are many causes of cancer, but dietary factors may have more to do with the development of more types of cancer than any other single factor. According to the Deputy Director of the National Cancer Institute, as quoted in Dietary Goals, "In the United States, the number of cancer cases a year that appear to be related to diet are estimated to be 40 percent of the total incidence for males and about 60 percent of the total incidence for females. The forms of cancer that appear to be dependent on nutrition as shown by epidemiologic studies include: Stomach, liver, breast, prostate, large intestine, small intestine, and colon."

Nutritional Deficiencies in Cancer

Colon cancer, a leading cause of cancer death, is believed to be caused largely by lack of adequate fiber in diets that contain too much refined carbohydrate. Such diets usually also contain too much fat, which has been linked to breast cancer as well as to colon cancer.

Poor diets that do not contain adequate natural carbohydrate are deficient in vitamins and other micro-nutrients that are normally associated with fiber-rich natural foods. According to the U.S. Department of Agriculture, "There is a small but growing body of data suggesting that chronic low-level intake of some nutrients is a factor in the incidence of cancer in man. There is evidence that vitamin deficiency plays a role in the occurrence of cancer of the oral cavity in the esophagus. Chronic vitamin B complex deficiency, due to inadequate supply of vegetables in the diet, appears to be incriminated." (*Human Nutrition,* Report No. 2.)

A deficiency in any vitamin or mineral can be a contributing factor in the development of cancer. Vitamins A and C, for example, are important in the construction of strong tissue that is resistant to invasion by germs and cancer cells. Vitamins C and E have anti-oxidant properties that protect cell membranes from the destructive effects of oxygen. Deficiencies in such trace minerals as zinc, selenium, and magnesium, which occur as a result of refining grains, may also contribute to the development of cancer.

Pitting Macro-Nutrient Foods Against Cancer

Whether you are overweight or not, it's important to pay close attention to what you eat. When you go on a low-calorie diet to reduce body fat, it's absolutely essential that you balance your diet with a wide variety of fresh, natural foods. Anyone can lose weight by eating less. The secret of *healthful* dieting, however, is food selection. You must supply your body with essential nutrients while cutting down on calorie intake. Your macro-nutrient diet takes all this into consideration. With the larger part of your energy nutrients coming from natural carbohydrate, you'll get the fiber you need along with trace minerals and other essential nutrients. Adequate fiber in your diet will speed emptying the waste matter from your colon, preventing conversion of bile acids to carcinogenic toxins.

For a longer, healthier life, make your macro-nutrient diet a lifetime diet. You need all the vitamins, minerals, and fiber you can get from a balanced diet of macro-nutrient foods if you want to maintain your body's resistance to cancer or any other disease. Don't just quit eating when you want to lose weight. Instead, make an effort to eat *properly.* Hypnotism and ear staples are not a safe substitute for knowledgeable dieting.

PUT A STOP TO THE EPIDEMIC OF DIABETES MELLITUS

When whole grains are processed to produce white flour and refined cereals, many nutrients are lost, including the trace minerals chromium and zinc. We've known for a long time that refined carbohydrates, including sugar, contribute to the development of diabetes by flooding the blood with glucose, thus overworking the pancreas. There is now some evidence to indicate that a *chromium deficiency* resulting from excessive consumption of refined carbohydrates also contributes to the development of diabetes. "It has been postulated that the decreasing ability to handle glucose with age may reflect chronic marginal intake of chromium throughout life," says the author of *Human Nutrition.*

Since the body needs zinc to produce insulin, a *zinc defi-*

ciency resulting from subsisting on refined carbohydrates may also contribute to the development of diabetes.

Because of dietary factors, *one out of every 20 Americans has diabetes or is potentially diabetic!*

Inability of the body to produce the insulin it needs to burn glucose for energy or to store it as glycogen results in such early warning signs as fatigue, frequent urination, excessive thirst, and loss of weight. (Sugar accumulating in the blood is eliminated by the kidneys instead of being used by the body.) Full blown diabetes results in abnormal fat metabolism that contributes to the development of vascular disease.

Handling Diabetes with Macro-Nutrient Foods

Diabetes in young people can be a hereditary disorder. But when it develops in adults, it may be caused (and controlled) by diet. Seven out of ten diabetics discover that they have the disease after age 45, indicating that diet may be a more common factor than heredity.

You already know from reading other chapters of this book that diabetics do well on a diet that is high in *natural* carbohydrates. So whether you're preventing diabetes or treating the disease, a macro-nutrient diet will serve you well. You should, of course, be under a physician's care if you have diabetes. But if you eliminate sugar, white flour, and other refined carbohydrates in your diet and include fiber-rich, nutrient-rich natural carbohydrates in a balanced diet, you may be able to avoid the use of insulin. Remember, however, that only a physician can diagnose diabetes. And whether you need insulin or not must be determined by blood tests.

HOW TO ADJUST YOUR DIET TO RELIEVE
GLUTEN ALLERGY

On a macro-nutrient diet in which 48 to 58 percent of your energy is derived from natural carbohydrates, your intake of whole grains will be generous. The bran supplied by grains provides most of the fiber that reaches your colon. Dietary fiber supplied by vegetables, fruits, and whole-grain products benefits your entire intestinal tract. But it's the crude fiber supplied by whole-grain products that survives the digestive process. So it's important to include all types of grains in your diet—unless you have a special problem.

If you happen to be allergic to *gluten*, a protein found in wheat, rye, oats, buckwheat, and barley, ingestion of these grains in any form will result in abdominal distension and diarrhea characterized by foamy, pale stools that contain a considerable amount of fat. Loss of fat-soluble vitamins and other nutrients through the stool can lead to anemia, soft bones, loose teeth, skin diseases, and other deficiency diseases.

Gluten allergy is called celiac disease. This disease is fairly rare and usually begins during the first year of life. Symptoms can appear, however, from age 20 to age 30. If you suffer from diarrhea in the form of light-colored stools, see a gastroenterologist.

How to Eliminate Gluten in Your Diet

Gluten is normally a healthful protein substance. But if your doctor tells you that you are suffering from celiac disease, you'll have to avoid wheat, rye, oats, barley, and other foods containing gluten. *This means that you cannot eat grains and their products except those made from corn and rice.* Flour made from corn, rice, arrowroot, soybeans, potatoes, artichokes, and gluten-free wheat starch can be used in cooking. You can purchase gluten-free bread in most health food stores. Whole-grain corn meal can be used to make a fiber-rich bread (see Chapter 6). Brown rice or hominy can be used as a cereal.

Remember that spaghetti, bread crumbs, macaroni, noodles and white flour are usually made from wheat. Milk shakes, beer, and other beverages containing malt (a barley extract) must also be avoided. Read the labels on the products you buy. Exclude those that contain "wheat flour." Canned meats and cold cuts, like many processed foods, sometimes contain a wheat product. Stick to fresh, natural foods. You'll have to avoid use of wheat bran, but you can substitute corn bran or rice bran, both of which have a higher crude fiber content than wheat bran.

HOW TO COMBAT DIVERTICULITIS WITH FIBER

Diverticulitis is a disease in which small pouches on the colon become inflamed to produce intestinal spasms that are accompanied by diarrhea or constipation. Pain is usually felt in the lower left portion of the abdomen. When a pouch becomes infected or clogged, it can rupture into the abdomen causing peritonitis.

About 30 percent of all persons over the age of 45 have diverticula (pouches) on their colon. The diagnosis of diverticulitis is not made, however, unless the diverticula become inflamed.

Doctors used to treat diverticulitis with a bland diet, instructing their patients to avoid foods containing fiber. Now we know that *lack* of adequate fiber in the diet results in the formation of pouches in the colon. When there is not enough fiber in the diet to sweep these pouches clean, they become clogged and inflamed. Diets high in protein, fat, and refined carbohydrate and low in fresh fruits, vegetables, and grains fill the colon with a heavy, tightly packed residue that clogs the colon and produces constipation. Then, when the colon contracts forcefully in a vain effort to empty the bowels, the waste is further packed into swollen pouches where rock-like impactions are formed. This results in inflammation, pain, spasm, and diarrhea.

Clean Your Colon with Food Brooms

It's now well known that the best way to treat or prevent diverticulitis is to increase your intake of fiber-rich foods. Adequate fiber in the colon holds water and keeps the stool light, soft, and bulky for easy elimination. (Portions of your stool will actually float when your diet is rich in fiber.) Even miller's bran, once rejected in the treatment of diverticulitis, can be used safely and effectively in relieving symptoms and sweeping out colon pouches.

In *acute* cases of diverticulitis where a pouch is infected or abscessed, a physician may prescribe bulk in the form of a special stool softener along with a special diet. It's important to make sure that no seeds or husks are ingested in order to avoid triggering a spasm that might rupture a swollen diverticulum. In *chronic* diverticulitis, a high-fiber diet made up largely of natural carbohydrates offers the best protection.

Everyone should avoid refined carbohydrates and low-carbohydrate diets that are so deficient in fiber that they produce chronic constipation. You won't have to worry about your bowels if at least half of your energy intake is supplied by complex (natural) carbohydrate. Score another plus for your macro-nutrient diet!

HOW TO AVOID GOUTY ARTHRITIS
ON A REDUCING DIET

Generally, gout is a genetic disorder in which the body produces an excessive amount of uric acid, or the kidneys may simply
be unable to eliminate uric acid. In either case, uric acid accumulating in the blood is deposited in joints and tissues in the
form of needle-like crystals, causing the swelling and inflammation
known as gouty arthritis.

The disease most commonly appears in the big toe, instep,
ankle, knee, wrist, and elbow. The affected joint is usually swollen
and throbbing with pain, and the overlying skin is hot, shiny, and
dusky red or purplish in color. The pain can be so excruciating and
the joint so sensitive that even the weight of the bed sheet is
intolerable.

Dietary Recommendations for Gout Victims

Dietary uric acid is formed from purines, which are found in
protein-rich foods such as meat, fish, poultry, beans, and wheat.
Gout patients are usually advised to get most of their protein from
milk, eggs, cheese, and other purine-free foods. Corn bread is
substituted for wheat bread, and so on. But since gout is often a
genetic disorder in which the body itself produces too much uric
acid, it's sometimes necessary to take special medication to help
the body dispose of the accumulating acid.

During an attack of gouty arthritis, it may be necessary to
increase your intake of fresh fruits, vegetables, and juices in order
to alkalize your urine and prevent the formation of uric acid stones.
You may also have to drink up to three quarts of water each day to
help your kidneys flush uric acid from your body.

Even if your doctor prescribes medication for your gout, you
should alter your diet to reduce your need for medication and to
help prevent recurring attacks. Testing your blood for uric acid will
reveal how well your body—and your diet—is handling the disease.

Actually, there is no cure for gout. Once the disease appears,
it must be kept under control with diet or medication—or both.

Reducing Diets and Gout

Overweight commonly accompanies gouty arthritis. If you are overweight, reducing your body weight will reduce your tendency to develop gout. But don't try to lose too much weight too fast. If weight loss is too rapid, an attack of gouty arthritis can be triggered by excessive burning of body fat (releasing uric acid). So if you are predisposed to gout, don't try to lose more than two or three pounds a week. Weight loss is more permanent anyway if it is gradual rather than rapid.

If you have never suffered an attack of gouty arthritis, don't worry about the purine content of meat and other protein-rich foods in a balanced diet. When body metabolism is normal and there is no genetic predisposition to gout, a good, balanced diet that includes meat will *not* cause gout. Persons who do suffer from gout, however, should go easy on meats and lean more toward a lacto-ovo-vegetarian type of diet (see Chapter 5).

Gouty arthritis is such a common complication of some low-carbohydrate, rapid weight loss diets that physicians who prescribe such diets may also routinely prescribe drugs to prevent a buildup of uric acid. Any drug is potentially harmful to your body. It doesn't make any sense at all to go on a diet so extreme or so low in calories that use of drugs becomes part of the diet, especially when there is a better way. And there *is* a better way! On a macro-nutrient diet in which at least one half of your energy intake is supplied by *natural carbohydrates,* your chances of developing gouty arthritis are slim or nonexistent.

FIGHT ARTHRITIS WITH GOOD HEALTH
AND A GOOD DIET

Just about everyone develops some form of arthritis at some time in life. And it's generally agreed that there is no cure for arthritis. But according to the Department of Agriculture's *Human Nutrition,* "All of the arthritic conditions appear to be associated with adverse changes in nutrient metabolism. The dietary changes needed to prevent or modify the severity of the arthritic condition are not known. There is a good possibility that research on the special nutrient requirements and food needs of persons predisposed to arthritis would yield great benefit to those likely to be affected."

There are, of course, many kinds of arthritis, but rheumatoid arthritis, gouty arthritis, and osteoarthritis are the most common. You have already learned in this chapter that although gouty arthritis is usually the result of an inherited metabolic disorder, you can often alleviate the disease by reducing your intake of foods that are rich in purine.

Rheumatoid arthritis is a chronic inflammatory disease affecting connective tissue in the body. Although no specific dietary factor has been associated with rheumatoid arthritis, victims of this disease have been observed to have a negative nitrogen and calcium balance. This may indicate poor absorption of protein and calcium.

In osteoarthritis, there is degeneration of the cartilage in the joints. "Heredity and diet are believed to be underlying factors," says *Human Nutrition.*

A Diet for Every Arthritic

What you eat may have something to do with the development or the severity of your arthritis, so it's important to make sure that your diet is nutritious and well-balanced, as in a macronutrient diet. Foods should be completely natural whenever possible. Too much sugar or refined carbohydrate in your diet, for example, might disturb calcium metabolism and create a deficiency in some of the B vitamins. You must include fruits in your diet to supply the Vitamin C you need for strong collagen in joint cartilage. The acid provided by fruits will aid absorption of protein, calcium, and iron.

Meats will supply the B vitamins you need for efficient body metabolism. But remember that too much meat might create an imbalance between calcium and phosphorus, resulting in a calcium deficiency. You must keep your diet balanced with selections from all four or seven basic food groups—to *prevent* arthritis as well as to *treat* arthritis. You can best reduce your body weight and meet the threat of arthritis by following a macro-nutrient diet in which 48 to 58 percent of your energy intake is supplied by natural carbohydrate. Food selections from *seven* basic food groups instead of four will assure a greater intake of fresh fruits and vegetables.

DEPENDING UPON THE WISDOM OF YOUR BODY

Although there is no known specific dietary cause or cure for arthritis, the better your diet the healthier your body and the less the chance that you'll develop a crippling form of arthritis. It's much better to supply your body with a variety of natural foods than to attempt to "balance body chemistry" by taking supplements. Only your body knows what it needs to function efficiently, and it must be provided with foods containing all the essential nutrients so that it can absorb what it needs. Everyone's needs are different. It's not possible to formulate supplements that will duplicate the combinations of nutrients absorbed from food, so don't ever be led to believe that you can replace a good, balanced diet with supplements.

Whether you're suffering from arthritis or any other disease, or you're only interested in preventing disease or reducing your body weight, you must make sure that your diet is balanced and healthful.

When Special Supplements Are Needed

When the body is diseased, or when deficiencies develop because of a bad diet or because of problems with absorption of nutrients, it may be necessary for a physician to prescribe special supplements. Persons who are deficient in stomach acid, for example, may have to take betaine hydrochloride tablets to aid absorption of calcium and iron. When the stomach is lacking in the intrinsic factor it needs to absorb Vitamin B_{12}, this vitamin must be injected to prevent the development of pernicious anemia. Intestinal diseases that result in loss of fat-soluble vitamins might require regular use of special supplements. Iron-deficiency anemia resulting from chronic bleeding or a poor diet must be corrected with iron supplements, and so on.

It's perfectly all right to take supplements for nutritional insurance. It's often necessary to take supplements to meet special needs or to correct deficiencies resulting from a bad diet or a diseased body. But the point is that *nothing* can substitute for a good diet in keeping your body healthy, especially when you are on a low-calorie diet. For this reason, *your macro-nutrient diet should be a lifetime diet*—to help protect against the development of disease as well as to keep you lean and physically attractive.

SUMMARY

1. *Your macro-nutrient diet will play an important role in preventing disease and protecting your health.*
2. *A diet high in natural carbohydrate will help prevent cardiovascular disease by increasing your intake of fiber and by reducing your intake of saturated fat and cholesterol.*
3. *Fresh, natural foods combined with regular exercise will help your body eliminate excess cholesterol by stimulating the formation of high-density lipoprotein in your blood.*
4. *A high-fiber, low-fat macro-nutrient diet will help prevent colon cancer, breast cancer, and a few other forms of cancer.*
5. *Chromium and other nutrients supplied by whole-grain products will help prevent diabetes.*
6. *In rare cases in which the intestinal tract is allergic to gluten, it may be necessary to avoid all whole-grain products except those made from corn and rice.*
7. *The best way to prevent and treat diverticulitis is to consume generous amounts of fiber-rich natural carbohydrates.*
8. *Persons predisposed to gouty arthritis must avoid rapid weight loss and go easy on such purine-rich foods as meats.*
9. *You can guard against the development of arthritis and other diseases by consuming a balanced diet that supplies your body with all the essential nutrients.*
10. *Except in cases of deficiency caused by disease or a bad diet, you should depend upon food to supply your body with the right combinations of macro-nutrients and micro-nutrients.*

10

Maintaining Good Health
and an Ideal Body Weight
with Macro-Nutrient Foods
and a New Life Style

When you get your weight down to a desirable level, you can prevent further weight loss simply by taking in a few more calories. You eat all the same foods you ate on your reducing diet—just a little more. If you are fairly active, you can take in about 15 calories for each pound of body weight without gaining weight. In order to keep your diet balanced and healthful, however, it's important to keep a hand on your fat-burner throttle by dividing your energy intake among the macro-nutrients so that 58 percent of your calories come from natural carbohydrate. Protein should supply 12 percent or more of your calories, with less than 30 percent coming from fat.

Everything you've learned up to now can apply to your maintenance diet. So don't stop eating properly prepared fresh, low-fat natural foods just because you're no longer fat. Remember that you're eating for good health as well as to maintain your ideal weight. *You should continue to eat that way as long as you live.*

After you have been counting calories for awhile on a macro-nutrient diet, you'll become familiar enough with the general nutrient value of natural foods to eat properly without actually measuring food portions. You'll develop dietary judgement and good eating habits that will stay with you for the rest of your life, thus improving the *quality* of your life.

The case of Roger C. provides a good example of how good eating habits can improve your life. When Roger was 95 pounds overweight, he spent most of his time sitting at home. "I just didn't feel like doing much," he explained. After Roger lost 90 pounds on a macro-nutrient diet, he experienced a surge of energy and confidence. "I look and feel so much better since I've reduced my body weight," Roger testified, "that I'm now doing more and enjoying it more. I'm even making more money because of my new look. I'm so proud of the way I look that I actually *enjoy* getting out to promote my business. Your macro-nutrient diet has really changed my life!"

YOU ARE UNIQUE

You should not be concerned about keeping your body weight at exactly the same weight given on a chart for someone of your height and frame. If your weight is near your ideal weight and you *look* good, it may not be necessary to deprive yourself on an extremely low-calorie diet just to lose a few more pounds. You can switch to a maintenance diet any time your physical appearance is pleasing to *you*.

It's important to understand that reaching your ideal body weight doesn't necessarily mean that your physical proportions will change. If you have unusually large calves or ankles, for example, they will probably remain disproportionately large even after all excess body fat is gone. So don't expect to be transformed into a "Miss America" or a "Mr. Universe" by a reducing diet. You'll look 100 percent better, of course, but if you want to change your body proportions you'll have to develop your muscles. See my book *Peter Lupus' Celebrity Body Book* (Parker Publishing Company) for special body-shaping exercises.

WHY YOU SHOULD INCLUDE EXERCISE
IN YOUR MAINTENANCE PROGRAM

It's always a good idea to take regular exercise, whether you're overweight or not. Exercise is especially helpful in reducing excess body fat, since it *forces* burning of stored fat for energy.

Most people who exercise regularly can lose weight *without* dietary restrictions. When exercise is *combined* with dietary restrictions, you can lose *twice* as much weight as you can by either measure alone. When exercise is included on a maintenance diet, you can take in considerably more calories than usual without gaining weight.

Even if you did not include exercise in your reducing program, chances are you'll want to begin exercising when all the excess fat is gone. You'll feel so much better at your lighter weight that you'll be naturally inclined to participate in some form of recreational activity such as swimming or tennis. Furthermore, you'll look so much better that you might want to get out and show off a little. In doing so, you'll burn enough calories to make your maintenance diet a snap.

The National Research Council recommends 2,400 calories daily for the average sedentary man and about 4,500 calories daily for *active* men. Athletes and some laborers may require as much as 6,000 calories a day to meet energy needs. Obviously, the more exercise you take the more you can eat on a maintenance diet. If you like to eat, you should take advantage of the effects of exercise when eating for pleasure.

Exercise Governs Appetite

If you don't like to exercise, don't excuse your inactivity by saying that exercise makes you overeat by increasing your appetite. Exercise will, of course, generate a healthy appetite. But if you exercise regularly, your calorie output will usually exceed your calorie intake. Inactivity, on the other hand, tends to increase the appetite abnormally, thus exceeding calorie needs. *Research has demonstrated that sedentary people tend to eat more than physically active people.* Inactivity combined with overeating is sure to result in a buildup of body fat.

Thus, all the available evidence indicates that if you take regular exercise you'll eat *less* than persons who do *not* exercise. Also, you'll be less likely to eat more than your body needs. One reason for this seems to be that exercise stimulates the body's metabolic processes so that the appetite mechanism in the brain functions more efficiently. This mechanism, called the appestat, regulates your appetite according to your body's needs. An inactive person eats to satisfy his stomach rather than his muscles and his brain. Body fat is stored as a result of inactivity as well as overeating, so even if you aren't overweight, *controlling your body weight on a maintenance diet can best be accomplished by combining diet and exercise in order to keep your appetite mechanism in good working order.*

Note: You can quell the sensation of hunger by exercising. When you use your muscles in vigorous physical activity, stored glycogen is converted to glucose and released for use as fuel. This results in an increase in blood sugar which satisfies the appetite mechanism in the brain. The next time you feel an irresistible urge to eat a forbidden food, you can relieve your misery by getting out and taking a little exercise.

Getting the Most for Your Effort

The endurance kinds of exercise such as tennis, swimming, or handball burn more calories and do more for your heart than other forms of exercise. But such simple exercise as gardening, dancing, or walking is better than nothing. You can burn 250 to 300 calories an hour gardening or walking. If you walk *briskly* for about 15 minutes each day, you can burn the equivalent of two pounds of body fat a year. Fast dancing can burn 500 to 600 calories an hour!

Any form of exercise that burns at least 10 calories a minute (600 calories an hour) will strengthen your heart as well as force burning of stored body fat. If you exercise regularly enough to work your way up to 20 minutes or more of continuous endurance exercise, you'll get the full benefit of exercise. But you must exercise at least every other day in order to stay in shape.

Burn Up to 15 Calories a Minute!

Table 10-1 shows the average number of calories burned per hour in a few popular physical activities. Pick something you like best. Remember that the heavier you are the more calories you'll burn per minute. (To figure calories per minute, divide 60 into the number of calories burned per hour.)

Endurance exercise should be worked into your schedule so that you can spend at least 10 minutes warming up for 20 minutes or more of exercise at least every other day.

Calories per Hour

Bowling	160-190
Walking (3 m.p.h.)	240-300
Softball	250-280
Golf (without cart)	240-320
Swimming	380-420
Bicycling (10 m.p.h.)	350-449
Tennis (singles)	420-480
Skiing (downhill)	500-590
Fast dancing	500-600
Skating (vigorously)	520-620
Jogging (5.5 m.p.h.)	600-660
Basketball	630-750
Handball	650-755
Skiing (cross country)	up to 1,000

Table 10-1

Walking Is Good Exercise

You can easily work walking into your daily schedule. If you drive a car to work, for example, you can park your car a couple of blocks away from your destination and walk the rest of the way. Instead of using an elevator, you can use the stairs. For best results, walk briskly. Climb stairs energetically. Walk *around* the block when you have the time. Make an extra trip up and down the stairs when you feel strong enough to do so. Walk or ride a bicycle to the neighborhood grocery store. Shop daily instead of once a week.

Anyone should be able to find enough time to walk or ride a bicycle for 15 minutes three or four times a day. With the price of gasoline skyrocketing, you can benefit financially as well as physically by acquiring the ability to walk rapidly for a mile or two. Walking is fashionable, and bicycles are "in." Be smart and get in step. Make walking and bicycling a part of your way of life.

Actor Joe Campanella gets all the exercise he needs by walking, playing ball with his boys, and performing chores around the house. To strengthen his arms and shoulders, he lifts his youngest children overhead several times a day. "My advice to anyone who wants to stay in shape is to do what you can to *stay active*," says Joe. "Walk more. Ride a bicycle. I run some, but I hate jogging. What I do is alternately sprint and walk. You can get adequate exercise simply by going up and down stairs. You should always walk instead of ride when you have a choice. The important thing is to do something that *you* can do and then do it *regularly*."

How Walter Ate Generously After Losing
32 Pounds in Two Months

Walter P. weighed 220 pounds at a height of five feet eleven inches. With his large frame, he should not have weighed more than 179 pounds. To maintain the lighter weight, his calorie intake would normally be around 2,685 calories a day.

"I like to eat," Walter admitted, "so I don't want to cut my food intake too much. If I could lose two or three pounds a week, I'd be happy."

To lose *three* pounds of body fat a week under ordinary conditions, Walter would have to reduce his energy intake to about 1,200 calories a day (see Chapter 3 for explanation). A loss of only *two* pounds a week would allow him to consume about 1,700 calories a day. "You have to take in fewer calories than you need to maintain your projected *ideal* weight in order to burn stored body fat," I explained to Walter. "The fewer calories you take in under your ideal weight requirement, the more weight you lose. Of course, exercise burns calories, and regular exercise can create a calorie deficit. If you want to lose more than two pounds a week without going below 1,700 calories, you'll have to exercise a little."

Walter chose to combine exercise with a 1,700-calorie diet. He walked an hour each day to burn about 400 calories. He burned 500 calories in the evening by bicycling for an hour. The exercise and diet together resulted in a loss of about four pounds of body fat a week. After two months, Walter had lost 32 pounds. He then raised his calorie intake to about 3,000 calories a day and cut his exercise to one hour. This allowed him to maintain his ideal weight on a generous diet. "The foods I'm allowed to eat on a macro-nutrient diet are delicious as well as filling," Walter says when explaining his dieting method. "After going on a macro-nutrient diet, I wouldn't think of trying another diet."

If you want to lose more than two or three pounds a week without cutting your food intake too drastically, you, too, might prefer to exercise a little. For each 500 calories you burn daily in physical activity (while on a controlled diet), you can lose an additional pound of body fat a week. Or, if you are on a maintenance diet and you want to eat more, you can add another 500 calories to your diet for each hour of exercise you take.

The Surprising Effects of Combining Diet and Exercise

Because of the effect of exercise, many active persons lose several pounds of fat a week on a diet that would normally result in a weight loss of only two or three pounds. There are many unpredictable variables in any reducing or maintenance diet. Susan T., for example, followed the same type of program that I recommended for Walter. According to calorie computations, Susan could expect to lose only about three pounds of body fat a week. Instead, *she lost five pounds the first week and an average of four pounds a week thereafter*. It took her only six weeks to lose 25 pounds. And this was on a generous diet of macro-nutrient foods.

So while you can usually calculate loss of body fat on a carefully controlled diet, no two people should expect exactly the same results in total weight loss. Some lose more and some less than others. Body water, fat metabolism, muscle tone, and other factors play a role in weight loss registered on scales. Water loss or water retention probably accounts for most drastic and unexplained differences in weight loss.

If you exercise at all, chances are you'll lose quite a bit more weight than someone on the same diet who doesn't exercise. One thing is sure—if you combine exercise with your maintenance diet, you'll be able to eat considerably more than you could otherwise.

Try to make daily recreational exercise a part of your life style. Exercise, like brushing your teeth, should be a health *habit*.

HOW TO MODIFY YOUR BEHAVIOR
TO MAKE DIETING EASIER

There are many factors that affect your eating habits. *When, where, why and how you eat,* for example, may have as much to do with overweight as inactivity or eating the wrong foods. If you habitually snack during coffee breaks at the office, you're eating for reasons other than to satisfy hunger or to meet your body's needs. If you eat while watching TV or while conducting business, you may be eating excessively without even being aware of your overindulgence.

How Lucy Lost 20 Pounds Simply by Modifying Her Behavior

Lucy R. complained that she could not lose weight on any kind of diet. "I've tried many diets," she explained, "and I never lost an ounce."

I asked Lucy to write down everything she ate for seven days. And I told her to note the time and location of her eating, even if she had only a bite. The results were eye opening. We discovered that Lucy had a habit of nibbling while talking and while watching morning and afternoon television. Gossipy telephone calls received in the kitchen were usually handled with one hand in the cookie jar. In attempting to record such snacks, Lucy was distressed to learn that she really did not know how much she ate. Because of the distraction of conversation or television, she could not re-member *what* she ate, much less how much.

"I had always thought that I could eat less at mealtime to make up for my snacks," Lucy observed. "But I can see now that I was eating without even being aware of what I was doing. I've been a compulsive, habitual snacker!"

Once Lucy realized what was happening, she was able to modify her behavior so that she could control her calorie intake. She limited her eating to mealtimes at the dining room table. She moved the telephone from the kitchen to the hall where she would have to stand to receive calls. No snacks were allowed in the television room. As a result of making these simple changes, Lucy started to lose weight—without counting calories.

"It's incredible how making a few changes in my behavior has made the difference in my weight," Lucy reported happily. "I'll never again eat while talking or while watching television."

Lucy lost 20 pounds of body fat in six months by doing nothing more than refusing to eat anything except when she was seated at the dining room table!

The rest of this chapter will be devoted to outlining a few behavior modification tips that *you* can follow to lose weight or to prevent weight gain—regardless of the type of diet you're on.

Eat Only at the Dining Room Table

When and where you eat can be as much a conditioned reflex as reaching for food when you are hungry. If you are accustomed to eating while watching television or while sitting in a theater, you might automatically reach for food everytime you sit down in front of your television set at home. Like Pavlov's dogs, which ate at the sound of a bell, you might develop conditioned reflexes that trigger a desire to eat as a result of environmental stimulation, even if you aren't hungry. For this reason, I usually advise my patients to eat only at the dinner table, at appointed times, without the distraction or the pleasure of television or movies. Don't allow yourself to become conditioned to eat everytime you are entertained.

Eating at the same time each day at the dinner table can also become a conditioned reflex. But you'll be eating more to satisfy hunger than for other reasons. And you'll be less likely to feel a desire to eat at other times during the day or night. Best of all, regular meals will contribute to good bowel habits and a more orderly way of life.

Try to schedule your eating at the dining room table where you can eat to meet the needs of your body rather than to satisfy a nervous habit. Avoid eating at movies. If you indulge your sense of pleasure to the hilt by stuffing your mouth while you're being entertained, you won't be able to separate eating from other forms of pleasure. You may then find it impossible to lose weight.

Eat Slowly and Chew Your Food Thoroughly

Many people eat so fast that they literally bolt their food without chewing it. The result is that they usually overeat. When you are truly hungry, a drop in sugar and other nutrients in your blood triggers an appetite mechanism in your brain, creating a desire for food. When you eat, it takes a little time (about 20 minutes) for your blood to absorb the needed nutrients and then circulate them to your brain where the sensation of hunger can be switched off. If you eat too rapidly, you may overload your stomach before your appetite mechanism has a chance to diminish your desire for food. If you eat slowly, however, chances are you'll experience satisfaction before you've had a chance to gobble down everything in sight.

You can prolong eating time by cutting your food into small bites and eating one bite at a time, chewing each bite thoroughly. Slices of bread can be cut into halves or quarters. Take time to taste and savor each bite. If you eat strictly natural foods, as you have been instructed to do, the foods you eat won't artificially stimulate your appetite. You'll quit eating when you have had enough.

Use Small Plates and Small Glasses

Serving your food on a small plate will help prevent overeating by limiting the size of food servings. If your plate appears to be full, it's easier to convince yourself that you're getting enough to eat. A large plate, however, will encourage overeating.

Even with a small plate, you should keep food portions small. Eat slowly. If you feel satisfied before all the food on your plate is gone, quit eating. Don't ever stuff yourself just to clean up your plate. It would be better to throw away a little food than to force your body to store it as fat.

When you eat at home, serve yourself in the kitchen and then take your plate to the dining room table to eat. You'll be less likely to eat second helpings if the food supply is beyond arm's reach.

Cook only as much food as you can eat in one day—or a little less. This way, you won't be tempted to overeat by finishing leftovers. Besides, it's always best to cook your foods fresh each day. Leftover food loses nutrients and is not as healthful as freshly prepared food.

Don't Conduct Business over Meals or Eat Meals at Parties

It's a common business practice to entertain prospective customers or clients by wining and dining them in exclusive restaurants. And in order to create the proper impression, it's customary to order rich, expensive meals, complete with cocktails. The result is that everyone involved is usually stuffed with high-calorie foods and beverages. Furthermore, when attention is focused on the business at hand rather than on meeting nutritional needs, eating becomes a social lubricant that serves only to calm nerves and to punctuate clever remarks.

It's nice to eat out occasionally. But if you have business to conduct, try to separate it from your eating so that you have full control over food selection as well as over when, where, why, and how you eat.

When you have to attend parties where food is served, eat your meals at home beforehand so that you can be sure of what you're eating. Then, if you like, you can save room for a light snack if you can find something that looks healthful. You can sip on Perrier water instead of alcohol or punch. Don't eat fattening foods or drink sweet drinks just to be sociable. If you have fat friends who are constantly badgering you to eat as they do, find new friends. Misery loves company. Some fat people who do not have the knowledge or the self-control to eat properly might feel threatened by examples of nutritional discipline.

If you have control of your life, you can eat the way you know you should eat, no matter what everyone else is eating.

Don't Use Food as a Tranquilizer

Eating to ease the misery of boredom, loneliness, or frustration is one of the major causes of overweight. Many people try to displace emotional distress with the pleasure of eating. The result is that eating becomes a nervous habit, like smoking cigarettes. When this happens, eating is no longer governed solely by your appetite mechanism but by forced reflex feeding. When my dog is mad, nervous, or excited, he runs to his bowl and eats as if he were starving. Many people do pretty much the same thing. But eating does no more to solve their problems than sticking their heads in the sand. What it really does is *add* to their problems by building up body fat.

It's always better to work off frustration or nervous tension by exercising rather than by turning to food. The depression accompanying boredom or loneliness will usually also disappear when body chemistry and circulation are stimulated by exercise. The rejuvenation that accompanies a few minutes of exercise can change your outlook from bad to good. Furthermore, thoughts about food will disappear when blood is diverted to your muscles. And when your liver releases glucose to provide fuel for your muscles, your appetite mechanism will switch to the "off" position. Best of all, you'll feel better—and you'll have an easier time maintaining a slim, youthful body.

Don't Allow Junk Food in Your Home

You know from reading earlier chapters of this book that refined-food snacks contain only empty calories. They also artificially stimulate your appetite, just as desserts do. Even when you say "I can't eat another bite," you can usually "make room" for a tasty snack or dessert.

Commercially prepared snacks are usually so tasty that they override your appetite mechanism, compelling you to eat for the sheer pleasure of taste. When such snacks are readily available, few people can resist them, much less eat only one small bite.

It's perfectly all right to eat an occasional snack or dessert that has been prepared at home to make sure that it is natural and nutritious. Even then, however, snacks and desserts should be eaten sparingly. *Commercial* snacks and desserts should be barred from your home.

You'll find it much easier to avoid buying junk food if you do your grocery shopping *after* you have eaten at home. When you are hungry and your blood sugar is low, packaged snacks, especially sweets, are difficult to resist.

Keep a supply of fresh fruit, raw vegetables, or popcorn on hand to satisfy an irresistible urge to snack. You can purchase healthful sweets in a health food store. But you must limit use of any type of sweets to only a few bites—and that requires considerable self-control. If you eat properly and keep your blood sugar under control, you'll find it much easier to resist sweets.

How to Handle Coffee Breaks

Whether you work at home or in an office, chances are you take a "coffee break." The idea of a midmorning and midafternoon break is to relieve fatigue or tension. Such relief is best obtained by lying down or by exercising, depending upon the type of work you're doing. If you sit most of the day, for example, you should spend your break walking or taking a little exercise. But if you perform physical labor, you should sit down and rest. In either case, a snack might be refreshing if it is wholesome and appropriate.

Athletes and other persons who work very hard physically might benefit from snacks that are designed to restore glycogen reserves. It's not likely, however, that the average person would expend enough energy between meals to lower the blood sugar. A snack between meals, therefore, usually provides unneeded calories. If you do have snacks between meals, you should take their calorie value into account when figuring your daily calorie needs.

Most people spend their coffee breaks eating junk foods supplied by commercial dispensers. You can make sure that your coffee-break snacks are healthful by carrying your own snacks. But you must also make sure that you take something that will fit in with your diet (see Chapter 8). You don't have to eat the doughnuts and other sweets that are passed around the office. You should not emulate the eating habits of friends and parents if they eat badly. Do what you have to do to eat the way that's best for you. If you eat like someone who's fat, chances are you'll be fat, too.

TAKE CHARGE OF YOUR LIFE

No matter how many diet books you read or how many doctors you go to, what you eat and how you take care of your body is *your* responsibility. You must learn how to eat properly and how to develop your life style so that weight control becomes a part of your way of life. If you must always depend upon someone to tell you exactly what to eat every time you need to lose weight, you won't succeed in keeping your weight down.

Study this book carefully. Read it again and again until you fully understand the principles of dieting. Then take charge of your life and your diet. Discipline yourself so that you work, eat, and sleep on a regular schedule. Keep up-to-date on nutrition by reading popular health magazines. Be the master of your body and your health.

Teresa Lost 45 Pounds—and Now Preaches Good Nutrition

When Teresa K. reduced her body weight from a burdensome 165 pounds to a breezy 120 pounds, she broke away from a lifestyle that lived and breathed fat. Teresa's parents were fat, and she had fat friends. Even her boyfriend was fat. Fat encouraged fat.

After Teresa's fat melted away on a macro-nutrient diet, her personality and her needs changed along with her figure. New eating habits were accompanied by new friends and new activities. "I no longer eat the way I used to eat," Teresa explained. "And I'm no longer ashamed to eat in public. In fact, I'm now proud of the way I eat. I'm constantly offering people advice on how to eat. I'm getting married soon, and I intend to pass my dietary knowledge along to my family. I don't want my children to be hindered by fat the way I was."

I can't think of a better gift for your family or your friends than to impart a little good advice on how to eat properly. If you make good use of this book, you can be a teacher of good nutrition as well as an example of good nutrition.

Keep Yourself Physically Attractive

Although you keep your body covered with clothing most of the time, how you look undressed can have a big impact on your life. If you have a fat or flabby body, for example, you may be as reluctant to undress for love as for a swim. "Having a good body is important," says comedian Paul Lynde. "I think the most guarded secret is what you think you look like nude. This results in many inhibitions. If I had a gorgeous body, I'd be nude all the time. A beautiful body is a beautiful thing to see, and it provides incentive to stay in shape rather than wear robes all the time. I think most people are ashamed of their bodies, so they hide in robes. I say if you've got it, flaunt it. I wear my robes when I take a shower."

When your body is lean and trim, you'll look just as good undressed as dressed. Half the battle of getting the weight off and keeping it off is feeling pleased with your physical appearance. This may mean exercising your muscles and tanning your skin as well as dressing smartly. If you take pride in your physical appearance, you'll pay more attention to your diet. So do all you can to *look* good. It's not vain to be body conscious. Keeping yourself physically attractive will pay big dividends in all phases of your life, especially your sex life.

Sex and Physical Appearance

Darlene R. complained about her husband's waning interest in sex. "My husband never looks at me anymore," Darlene confided tearfully, "and we rarely make love. I realize I'm overweight, but my husband says he likes me the way I am."

I told Darlene to quit kidding herself. Flabby fat is *never* attractive, especially when it comes to sex. I advised her to go ahead and reduce her body weight and see what effect it would have on her husband's attitude. The result was just as I had expected.

"Ever since I shed 45 pounds of fat," Darlene reported, "my sex life has been getting better and better. My husband is so turned on by the way I look that we have returned to the sexual preliminaries we used to enjoy so much. It's like a new, *better* honeymoon. Don't tell anyone I told you this, but my husband has actually installed mirrors in our bedroom. And to tell you the truth, *I* like the way I look, too."

How *you* look can have much to do with how much you enjoy life—in or out of bed! The macro-nutrient diet outlined in this book will improve your physical appearance as well as your health. You can't ask for more than that.

How Roxie and Hugh Regained Happiness by Losing Weight

Roxie and Hugh D. were lean and fit tennis players when they were married. Within months after their wedding ceremony, however, both of them were 20 pounds heavier. After one year of married bliss, the honeymoon was over. Roxie and Hugh were so fat and flabby that neither found the other attractive. Like many newly married couples, Hugh concentrated on earning a living while Roxie kept house and prepared meals. Eating for pleasure soon replaced sex, tennis, and other activities. The fatter Roxie and Hugh became the more they ate.

Finally, with Roxie weighing 170 pounds and Hugh tipping the scales at 230 pounds, a friend told them about macro-nutrient dieting. Doing nothing more than following general rules of proper eating (Chapter 1), Roxie reduced her weight to 125 pounds, only two pounds more than she weighed on her wedding day. Hugh shed 50 pounds, eliminating the jello-like fat on his body.

Roxie and Hugh once again found each other physically appealing. "We're reliving our honeymoon," they beamed. "And to make sure that our honeymoon doesn't end, we've changed our eating habits and joined the local spa."

If you want your life on earth to be one long honeymoon, be sure to modify your behavior as necessary to assure continuation of good eating habits. It's your life, and there's only one time around. So do all you can to grab all the "gusto" you can get. Don't let fat deprive you of your fair share of good living!

SUMMARY

1. *Your maintenance diet should be the same as your reducing diet—except that you just eat a little more.*
2. *You'll probably eat less if you exercise regularly than if you are sedentary, but the more exercise you take the more you can eat.*
3. *Recreational exercise and other forms of physical activity should be as much a part of your way of life as brushing your teeth.*
4. *When, where, why, and how you eat can have as much to do with overweight as eating the wrong foods.*
5. *Eating to supply the nutrients your body needs should not be artificially stimualted by combining eating with other forms of pleasure, such as watching television.*
6. *Use small plates and glasses to reduce the size of food servings and then eat only at the dining room table.*
7. *Always eat slowly, one bite at a time, in order to give your appetite mechanism time to reduce your desire for food.*
8. *Try to avoid the ceremony of eating meals while conducting business or attending parties.*
9. *When you feel bored, lonely, depressed, or frustrated, use exercise rather than food to relieve your distress.*
10. *Keeping yourself physically attractive will encourage good eating habits as well as contribute to a better life.*

11

Everyday Macro-Nutrient Menus
for Better Health
and a Slimmer Body

Generally, I do not recommend following a diet that tells you exactly what to eat at every meal. It's important, of course, to include food selections from all the basic food groups. But you should be able to eat the foods you like best in each group. If doesn't matter, for example, whether you eat lean meat, chicken, or fish as long as your diet is balanced to provide the iron and other micro-nutrients you need for good health. You can drink skim milk or you can eat cottage cheese for calcium. Practically any fresh fruit is suitable. Whole-grain products can be eaten in the form of bread or as cereals, and so on.

For a healthful reducing diet, it's important to make sure that the macro-nutrients (carbohydrate, protein, and fat) are consumed in correct proportions in order to supply your body with all the essential micro-nutrients without an oversupply of energy nutrients. To do this, you must balance your diet with *natural* foods from all the basic food groups and then make an effort to avoid sugar, white flour, and other refined foods as much as possible. Foods must also be properly prepared. Fat should be kept to a minimum by eliminating visible fats and by cooking without grease or oil.

Obviously, there is more to healthful reducing than just controlling your calorie intake. So be sure to make good use of all that

you have learned about fiber, food preparation, and behavior modification in developing your diet.

This chapter will provide you with a brief summary of how to
go on a macro-nutrient diet. But remember that *a macro-nutrient
diet is more than a reducing diet;* it's also a health-building,
disease-preventing diet. This is one reason why the new macro-
nutrient diet is probably the *best* diet you'll ever find. This diet will
change your eating habits, thus changing your life. And the diet
and its effects will last a lifetime.

You should periodically review every chapter of this book in
order to continue eating properly—whether you are overweight or
not.

PICK THE DIET PLAN THAT SUITS YOU BEST

Since I feel that the best reducing diet is one that allows you
to select the foods you like best from the basic food groups, I'll
outline a few basic diets that will allow you to choose your favorite
foods in the amounts you need to meet your particular calorie
requirements. Then I'll outline a few sample menus listing the
foods I would select. With such general guidance, you should be
able to make up your own menus with no trouble at all. But first
let's review the basic steps you must take to devise an effective
custom-made macro-nutrient diet.

FOLLOW THIS THREE-STEP APPROACH
TO A MACRO-NUTRIENT DIET

These three steps are covered in greater detail in Chapters 2
and 3. Turn back if you need additional information.

Step 1: First Determine Your Calorie Requirement

Most doctors simply issue a standard 1,200 calorie diet to
everyone who wants to lose weight. If you have a tall, large frame,
however, you can lose weight on a higher-calorie diet, maybe 1,800
calories or more. Of course, the fewer calories you consume, the
faster your weight loss. But it's important to make sure that you
supply your body with adequate nutrients. This usually means
keeping the rate of weight loss down around two to four pounds a
week.

If you are a large person, you'll have to eat more than a smaller person to keep your body healthy while losing weight. So not everyone can go on a 1,200 calorie diet safely. Besides, most of us want to be able to eat generously while we're losing weight. The best way to do this is to determine how much you can eat and still lose three or four pounds a week. You can control your reducing power pedal to suit yourself.

As a rule, a fairly active person who is not overweight can maintain an ideal weight by taking in about 15 calories for each pound of body weight each day. (See Chapter 3 for variations in requirements.) Find your ideal weight by consulting the height-weight chart in Chapter 3. Then multiply that weight by 15 to get your normal calorie requirement.

To lose one pound of body fat a week, subtract 500 calories from your normal *daily* calorie requirement. For each additional 500 calories you subtract daily, you can lose an additional pound of body fat a week. Remember that to burn *stored* body fat, you must take in fewer calories than you need to maintain your *ideal* weight. But you must make sure that you never take in fewer than 1,200 calories a day.

Step 2: Make Food Selections from the Basic Food Groups

Once you have determined how many calories you must take in to allow a desired rate of weight loss, you must make food selections from each of the basic food groups. Select the foods you like best. Make sure that your daily diet supplies at least two cups of skim milk or their equivalent in milk products (one ounce of cheese can be substituted for one cup of milk); two or more three-ounce servings of fish, poultry, or lean meat; three or more servings of vegetables with at least one serving of fruit; and four or more servings of whole-grain bread or cereal. See Chapter 2 for more information about the basic food groups.

Selections from *all* the basic food groups will assure a balanced intake of vitamins and minerals. Since vegetables, fruits, and whole-grain products are carbohydrates, using the *seven* basic food groups as a guide will make sure that at least half of your energy intake is supplied by carbohydrate. Of course, all foods must be fresh, natural, and prepared without fat, sugar, or white flour.

**Step 3: Check the Calorie and Nutrient Value
of Food Selections**

On a low-calorie diet (less than 2,000 calories), carbohydrate should not supply more than about 48 percent of energy intake in order to allow an intake of at least 60 grams of protein (22 percent of energy intake). Fat should *never* supply more than 30 percent of energy intake.

On higher calorie diets, especially maintenance diets, natural carbohydrates should supply about 58 percent of energy intake, leaving 12 percent for protein and 30 percent for fat. See Chapter 2 for details on figuring these percentages. The Table of Nutritive Values in the next chapter lists the weight of foods in grams and then breaks this weight down into grams of carbohydrate, protein, and fat. So it won't be difficult to determine the percentage of carbohydrate, protein, and fat in a food serving.

Fortunately, you don't have to be exact in figuring calories and percentages. Once you determine your calorie needs and then select from the basic food groups in supplying a certain number of calories, you'll come pretty close to getting the correct percentage of the macro-nutrients. As long as you're in the ball park, you're in the game.

As a rule of thumb, *your diet should supply about twice as many fruits, vegetables, and whole-grain products as meat and dairy products, with visible fats kept to a minimum.* With a little arithmetic, however, you can alter food selections to provide you with the best possible balance of macro-nutrients for healthful weight loss. You'll be able to control your fat-burner throttle with the skill of a pilot.

THE SPECIAL BENEFITS OF A MACRO-NUTRIENT DIET

Unlike most reducing diets, *everything you eat on a macro-nutrient diet is fresh and natural.* No refined or processed foods are allowed. Some reducing diets allow such foods as frankfurters and buns, cole slaw with mayonnaise, flour-thickened sauces, sugar-sweetened catsup, and other processed or concentrated foods. Such foods are so high in calories that they greatly reduce the volume of food allowed on a 1,200 calorie diet. A tablespoon of salad dressing supplying 55 calories, for example, can displace a piece of fruit or a couple of servings of fresh vegetables. The fruit and vegetables would do more to fill your stomach than a tablespoon of dressing—and they would supply more nutrients. Fruits and vegetables must, of course, be *fresh*. Canned vegetables, in addition to being deficient in nutrients, might actually contain sugar! It's important to stick to the basic idea of a macro-nutrient diet and eat fresh, natural foods that are properly prepared. Remember that even if a processed food does not contain many calories, it might be deficient in essential nutrients and loaded with harmful additives.

Benefits Experienced by Katrina D.

It has been my observation that a 1,200 calorie macro-nutrient diet is far superior to a 1,200 calorie diet that allows consumption of refined or processed foods. Consider the experience of Katrina D., for example. Katrina was trying to lose 30 pounds on a 1,200 calorie diet she had clipped from a popular magazine. She had lost a few pounds in three weeks on the diet, but she complained of fatigue, hunger, constipation, and a "rumbling, empty stomach."

When Katrina switched to the 1,200 calorie diet outlined in this chapter, all of her problems disappeared. Why? Because the fresh, natural foods in a macro-nutrient diet normalized her blood sugar, filled her stomach with a greater volume of food, and provided the fiber she needed to keep her bowels healthy and active. "I lost 28 pounds in nine weeks," Katrina reported with a radiant smile. "The nutrients I'm getting must be helping, because I'm feeling so energetic that I've taken on a part-time job in a dress shop. And believe it or not, I've even been doing a little modeling."

A New Life for Nick Z.

Big Nick Z. also experienced dramatic benefits on a macronutrient diet. Nick lost 150 pounds on a series of macro-nutrient diets that were adjusted down from 2,500 calories to 1,500 calories as weight loss progressed. This allowed Nick to lose weight without starving. "A macro-nutrient diet is the only way to go," Nick says enthusiastically. "Not only am I looking better and feeling better; my feet and my back have quit hurting. It's great to be able to play a game of tennis without feeling 90 years old. And I really like being able to tuck my shirt over a flat stomach."

Like many people who switch to a macro-nutrient diet, Nick experienced some additional special benefits. "I haven't had a headache since going on your diet," he said, "and my blood cholesterol has dropped nearly to normal."

Eliminating such foods as frankfurters and buns from his diet had eliminated cholesterol-building fats and refined carbohydrates as well as sodium nitrate and other additives that commonly cause headache and other symptoms.

You, too, will experience special benefits on a macro-nutrient diet. No other diet can do so much for your weight and your health. That's what makes this diet so special.

Use Sample Diets as a Guide in Developing Your Own Diet

This chapter will outline a few sample *basic* diets that supply from 1,200 to 2,500 calories. You can control your reducing power pedal by picking a diet that meets your calorie requirement for reducing or for maintaining body weight. Pick the foods you like best in making up your diet, but make sure that you include the types of foods given as examples.

You can easily adjust the calorie content of these diets by reducing or by increasing the size of food servings as needed. You can check the calorie content of food selections by referring to the Table of Nutritive Values in the next chapter.

All of the diets and menus in a macro-nutrient diet consist of basic, natural foods. No recipes or foods calling for the use of sugar, fat, or white flour are used. In addition to being lower in calories and more healthful, such a diet plan allows you to eat considerably *more* than if refined foods were included.

First I'll outline diet *plans* that will tell you what type of foods to eat. Then I'll outline sample *menus* listing specific examples of recommended foods.

A RAPID WEIGHT-LOSS 1,200+
CALORIE BASIC DIET PLAN

This diet plan supplies approximately 1,200 calories with about 120 grams of carbohydrate and 80 grams of protein. Bran has been added to provide filling bulk. If you still feel that your stomach is not full enough, drink a glass of water before each meal. A cup of bouillon between meals will help reduce your appetite by soothing the appetite mechanism in your brain. You may also snack on raw vegetables if you like.

Remember that diets supplying less than 2,000 calories should be supplemented with multiple vitamins and minerals.

Generally, I recommend 1,200 calorie diets for women and 1,500 calorie diets for men.

Breakfast

1 piece fresh fruit
1 slice whole-grain bread topped with one egg—*or*—1 serving of whole-grain cereal mixed with 1 tablespoon of miller's bran
1 cup skim milk
Unsweetened coffee if desired
Note: You may alternate the egg and the cereal so that you have three eggs a week.

Lunch

3 ounces chicken or fish
½ cup cooked vegetable
Green salad with vinegar dressing
1 slice whole-grain bread with pat of butter or margarine
1 piece fresh fruit
Water or unsweetened tea

Dinner

4 ounces chicken or fish
2 cooked vegetables, ½ cup each—*or*—1 cooked vegetable and a raw salad
1 slice whole-grain bread
1 piece fresh fruit
Water (with lemon or lime juice if desired) or vegetable juice

Bedtime Snack

1 tablespoon milk-moistened miller's bran
1 cup skim milk or ½ cup cottage cheese
Note: Moistened bran may be chewed and then washed down with milk or water.

SLOWER WEIGHT LOSS ON A 1,500+
CALORIE DIET PLAN

Most people (especially men) can lose weight on a 1,500 to
1,800 calorie diet if they are physically active. Determine your
calorie needs by comparing your existing weight with your ideal
weight and then adjust your diet accordingly for reducing or for
maintenance. Simply eating more vegetables, fruits, and whole-
grain products will increase your calorie intake without supplying
an excessive amount of fat. You need only about 15 to 25 grams of
dietary fat daily to provide essential fatty acids and to serve as a
carrier for fat-soluble vitamins. Otherwise, there is no specific requirement for fat as a nutrient in your diet.

Breakfast

6 ounces fruit juice
1 serving whole-grain cereal with diced fruit and 1 tablespoon
raisins and 1 tablespoon miller's bran—*or*—1 slice whole-grain
bread topped with one egg and 1 slice of whole-grain bread with 1
pat of butter or margarine
1 piece fresh fruit
1 cup skim milk
Unsweetened coffee if desired

Lunch

3 ounces lean meat, chicken, or fish
2 cooked vegetables, ½ cup each
Green salad with lemon juice dressing
2 slices whole-grain bread
1 piece fresh fruit
Water or unsweetened tea

Dinner

3 ounces lean meat, chicken, or fish
2 cooked vegetables, ½ cup each
Green salad with vinegar or lemon juice dressing
2 slices whole-grain bread
1 pat of margarine
1 piece fresh fruit
Water or vegetable juice

Bedtime Snack

1 cup skim milk or 1 ounce hard cheese
1 slice whole-grain bread
Note: Fruit allowed with meals can be reserved for between-meal snacks if desired. It takes a lot of food to supply 1,500 calories on a macro-nutrient diet. Persons not accustomed to eating three balanced meals a day might not feel comfortable eating so much at one meal.

BODY MAINTENANCE WITH A 2,500+
CALORIE DIET PLAN

If a 2,500 calorie diet fits your body size, weight, and activity level, you'll have *more* than enough to eat if you keep fat at a minimum and avoid sugar, commercial sweets and snacks, white-flour products, and other refined foods. In fact, if your weight is normal and you exercise regularly, you can eat just about anything you want that is fresh, natural, and low in fat. You can eat more natural sweets, such as dried fruits, honey, and natural ice cream. But don't eat any more than you need to satisfy your appetite. Stop eating when you feel that you've had enough, even if there is food left over. Just make sure that you eat some of *all* the basic foods.

Breakfast

Fruit juice
2 slices whole-grain bread
1 egg with 1 ounce lean meat
Whole-grain cereal with raisins and diced fruit
1 cup skim milk
Coffee if desired

Snack

Fresh Fruit

Lunch

4 ounces lean meat, chicken, or fish
2 cooked vegetables, ½ cup each
Raw vegetable salad with 1 tablespoon dressing
2 slices whole-grain bread
1 ounce dried fruit
Water or tea

Snack

½ cup uncreamed cottage cheese
1 piece fresh fruit

Dinner

4 ounces lean meat, chicken, or fish
2 cooked vegetables, ½ cup each
1 green salad with 1 tablespoon dressing
2 slices whole-grain bread
1 pat of margarine
1 cup skim milk
½ cup yogurt with fresh or dried fruit

Snack (Optional)

1½ ounce hard cheese with 1 slice whole-grain bread—*or*—2 tablespoons unhydrogenated peanut butter on 1 slice whole-grain bread.

Calories Are Essential

Persons who don't like to eat might ask "Why should I eat so
much if I'm not hungry or overweight?" It's just as important to eat
to obtain essential nutrients and to maintain a healthy body weight
as it is to avoid overweight. If your body is thin and you burn more
calories each day than you take in, chances are your health will
suffer. So don't ignore your diet just because you're not fat. You
must eat something from all the basic food groups each day if you
want to stay healthy and live a long time. If your scales or your
mirror begin to show a buildup of body fat, you should then begin
cutting back on the amount of food you eat. Use the height-weight
chart in Chapter 3 to figure your calorie needs.

SAMPLE BASIC MENUS FOR EVERYONE

It's difficult to be absolutely sure of how many calories you're
taking in unless you list specific foods in measured amounts. Beans,
for example, contain more calories than cabbage. Beef contains
considerably more calories than fish, and so on. Following the basic
diet plans outlined earlier will give you a general idea of your
calorie intake if you eliminate visible fat and cook without grease or

oil. But until you list your favorite foods in these diets, you won't have full control over your reducing power pedal.

Following are a few sample menus listing examples of foods *I* would select.

Basic 1,200 Calorie Menu

This sample menu clearly demonstrates that you can eat a lot of food on a 1,200 calorie diet if you stick to fresh, natural foods.

Breakfast

1 orange
1 egg
1 slice whole-wheat bread
1 pat of butter
1 cup skim milk
1 tablespoon milk-moistened miller's bran
Unsweetened coffee if desired

Lunch

3 ounces baked chicken
½ cup cooked carrots
Green salad
1 slice whole-wheat bread
1 pat of margarine
1 apple
Water or unsweetened tea

Dinner

6 ounces baked chicken
½ cup steamed cabbage
½ cup cooked carrots
Green salad with vinegar dressing
1 slice whole-wheat bread
1 banana
1 glass tomato juice

Bedtime Snack

1 cup skim milk
1 tablespoon milk-moistened miller's bran

Note: You can eat generous amounts of such vegetables as lettuce and tomatoes in a raw salad. Allotted fruits can be eaten between meals. If fats are kept to a minimum and refined carbohydrates are avoided, you'll have plenty to eat on a 1,200 calorie diet.

Basic 1,500 Calorie Menu

This menu has been a popular reducing diet for men.

Breakfast

2 shredded wheat biscuits
1 cup skim milk
½ banana and ½ apple diced into cereal
1 tablespoon raisins in cereal
1 slice whole-wheat bread
1 pat of butter
Coffee or Sanka if desired

Lunch

1 lean lamb chop, broiled
1 cup snap green beans
1 ear sweet corn
1 slice whole-wheat bread
1 pat margarine
Mixed raw-vegetable salad with lemon juice dressing
1 raw peach
Water or tea

Dinner

6 ounces broiled fish
1 medium baked potato
½ cup cut broccoli, cooked
Mixed raw-vegetable salad with lemon juice dressing
1 slice whole-wheat bread
1 pat of butter
¼ cantaloupe
Water or vegetable juice (V8)

Bedtime Snack

1 cup skim milk
1 slice whole-wheat bread

Basic 2,500 Calorie Maintenance Menu

Some of the foods allowed in this menu are higher in calories than the foods listed in the previous menus. One reason for this is to permit you to get the calories you need without overfilling your stomach. You may even have a little natural ice cream and other wholesome desserts—provided, of course, that you can eat them without gaining weight. *It's important, however, to continue eating fresh, natural foods, keeping fat at a minimum.*

Once you develop good eating habits, chances are your body weight won't seesaw and unwanted fat won't return. Remember, though, that if you habitually take in more calories than you need, you'll gain weight. So be sure to adjust your calorie intake according to your height, frame, and activity level.

Breakfast

1 glass (6 ounces) orange juice
1 egg
1 slice bacon
1 cup oatmeal with 1 tablespoon honey
1 slice whole-grain bread
1 pat margarine
1 cup skim milk
Coffee if desired

Snack

1 apple

Lunch

3 ounces lean pork
1 medium sweet potato
½ cup collards
Mixed raw vegetable salad with 1 tablespoon dressing
2 slices whole-wheat or corn pone
2 dried figs
Tea with 1 teaspoon sugar or honey

Snack

½ cup uncreamed cottage cheese with ⅓ cup fresh strawberries

Dinner

3 ounces lean round steak
½ cup asparagus
½ cup lima beans
2 slices whole-wheat bread
Mixed raw vegetable salad with 1 tablespoon dressing
1 cup skim milk
½ cup unsweetened applesauce

Snack

2 tablespoons unhydrogenated peanut butter on 1 slice whole-wheat bread
½ cup skim milk

USE COMMON SENSE AND IMAGINATION

Fresh, low-fat natural foods are so much lower in calories than refined foods that you might actually find it difficult to eat all the food allowed in your meals. Whenever this is the case, it would be better to eat smaller portions than to eliminate a basic food. You may also reserve some of your allotted foods for between-meal snacks.

You can be flexible in your eating when you are knowledge-able enough about food to switch or combine food selections in a balanced diet. You may occasionally convert a salad into a complete meal, for example, by mixing in such foods as tuna fish and cottage cheese.

Remember that the diet plans and menus outlined in this chapter are simply guides. You may select the foods you like best as long as your diet supplies the right number of calories and the correct percentages of energy nutrients (48 to 58 percent natural carbohydrate, 12 to 22 percent protein, and *never* more than 30 percent fat). You can easily make these determinations by using the Table of Nutritive Values in the next chapter.

You should, of course, eat a variety of foods during the week, with something from each of the basic seven food groups each day. But it's perfectly all right to have the same foods at dinner that you prepared for lunch. Few of us would attempt to eat completely different foods in all three meals every day of the week. This would result in waste as well as added expense. So use a little common sense when preparing meals at home.

If you study every chapter of this book, you'll know how to eat and how to diet. You'll be able to develop a diet plan that's best for you. Eating will be a challenge and an adventure as well as a pleasure.

SUMMARY

1. *On a macro-nutrient diet, you can select the foods you like best in the basic food groups.*
2. *Your calorie needs should be determined by comparing your existing weight with your ideal weight.*
3. *After you have decided how many calories you need and how fast you want to lose weight, you can select an appropriate diet plan.*
4. *Even on a maintenance diet, you should continue to eat fresh, natural foods, avoiding refined carbohydrates and keeping fat to a minimum.*
5. *On a fast weight-loss 1,200 calorie diet, you can use raw vegetables, miller's bran, and water to top off a partially filled stomach.*
6. *The calorie content of a basic 1,200+ calorie diet can be increased by adding more vegetables, fruits and whole-grain products.*
7. *Most people can lose weight slowly on a 1,500 calorie diet that is balanced with basic foods.*
8. *Lean, active persons often need 2,500 calories or more to maintain a healthy body weight.*
9. *For best results, your macro-nutrient diet must be tailored to your needs.*
10. *A macro-nutrient diet can be used to build and maintain health as well as to control body weight.* Be sure to continue using this book as a guide to eating, whether you're overweight or not.

12

Energy Nutrient Values
of Common Carbohydrate, Protein,
and Fat Macro-Nutrient Foods

It should be clear by now that macro-nutrient foods are simply fresh, natural foods that supply your body with the right combinations of vitamins, minerals, carbohydrate, protein, and fat. On a macro-nutrient diet, you operate your *reducing power pedal* by controlling your calorie intake. You adjust your *fat-burner throttle* by keeping the macro-nutrients (carbohydrate, protein, and fat) in proper proportions.

The Table of Nutrient Values in this chapter lists the calorie and macro-nutrient values of the types of foods allowed in your diet. Since a macro-nutrient diet does not recommend consumption of refined and processed foods, none are listed in the Table.

If you'd like to have a complete list of all types of foods, including processed foods, showing macro-nutrient and micro-nutrient (vitamins and minerals) values, you can order one from the U.S. Government Printing Office. Just write the Superintendent of Documents, U.S. Government Printing Office, Washington, D.C. 20402, and ask for *Nutritive Value of Foods*, Home and Garden Bulletin No. 72, or *Nutritional Value of American Foods in Common Units*, Agriculture Handbook No. 456.

REPORT YOUR RESULTS TO ME

I'd be interested in hearing from you after you have read this book and tried my macro-nutrient method of dieting. Reporting the results of your dieting to me will help compile the material I need for additional dietary research. Write to me, Dr. Samuel Homola, 609 N. Cove Blvd., Panama City, Florida 32401.

Best wishes for healthful, successful dieting!

Samuel Homola

TABLE OF MACRO-NUTRIENT VALUES*

	Weight Grams	Energy Calories	Protein Grams	Fat Grams	Carbohydrate Grams
Dairy Products					
Cheese:					
Cheddar, cut pieces, 1 oz	28	115	7	9	Trace
1 cu in	17.2	70	4	6	Trace
Cottage (curd not pressed down):					
Creamed (4% fat):					
Large curd, 1 cup	225	235	28	10	6
Small curd, 1 cup	210	220	26	9	6
Low fat (2%), 1 cup	226	205	31	4	8
Low fat (1%), 1 cup	226	165	28	2	6
Uncreamed (less than ½% fat)					
1 cup	145	125	25	1	3
Mozzarella, made with-					
Whole milk, 1 oz	28	90	6	7	1
Part skim milk, 1 oz	28	80	8	5	1
Ricotta, made with-					
Whole milk, 1 cup	246	428	28	32	7
Park skim milk, 1 cup	246	340	28	19	13
Swiss, 1 oz	28	105	8	8	1
Milk:					
Whole (3.3% fat), 1 cup	244	150	8	8	11
Lowfat (2%):					
No milk solids, added, 1 cup	244	120	8	5	12
Lowfat (1%):					
No milk solids added, 1 cup	244	100	8	3	12
Nonfat (skim):					
No milk solids added, 1 cup	245	85	8	Trace	12
Buttermilk, 1 cup	245	100	8	2	12

*Adapted from *Nutritive Value of Foods* (1978), U.S. Government Printing Office, Washington, D.C. 20402.

TABLE OF MACRO-NUTRIENT VALUES (continued)

	Weight Grams	Energy Calories	Protein Grams	Fat Grams	Carbo-hydrate Grams
Yogurt:					
With added milk solids:					
Made with lowfat milk:					
Plain, 8 oz	227	145	12	4	16
Made with nonfat milk:					
Plain, 8 oz	227	125	13	Trace	17
Without added milk solids:					
Made with whole milk:					
Plain, 8 oz	227	140	8	7	11

Eggs

Eggs, large:					
Raw:					
Whole, without shell, 1 egg	50	80	6	6	1
White, 1 white	33	15	3	Trace	Trace
Yolk, 1 yolk	17	65	3	6	Trace
Cooked:					
Fried in butter, 1 egg	46	85	5	6	1
Hard-cooked, shell removed	50	80	6	6	1
Poached, 1 egg	50	80	6	6	1

Fats and Oils

Butter:					
Regular:					
1 tbsp (about ⅛ stick)	14	100	Trace	12	Trace
1 pat	5	35	Trace	4	Trace
Whipped:					
1 tbsp	9	65	Trace	8	Trace
1 pat	4	25	Trace	3	Trace
Margarine:					
Regular:					
1 tbsp (about ⅛ stick)	14	100	Trace	12	Trace
1 pat	5	35	Trace	4	Trace
Whipped:					
1 tbsp	9	70	Trace	8	Trace
Oils, salad or cooking:					
Corn, 1 tbsp	14	120	0	14	0
Olive, 1 tbsp	14	120	0	14	0
Safflower, 1 tbsp	14	120	0	14	0

TABLE OF MACRO-NUTRIENT VALUES (continued)

	Weight Grams	Energy Calories	Protein Grams	Fat Grams	Carbo-hydrate Grams
Salad dressings:					
French, regular 1 tbsp	16	65	Trace	6	3
Italian, regular, 1 tbsp	15	85	Trace	9	1
Mayonnaise, 1 tbsp	14	100	Trace	11	Trace
Thousand Island, regular, 1 tbsp	16	80	Trace	8	2

Fish, Shellfish, Meat, Poultry

	Weight Grams	Energy Calories	Protein Grams	Fat Grams	Carbo-hydrate Grams
Fish and Shellfish:					
Bluefish, baked with butter, 3 oz	85	135	22	4	0
Clams:					
Raw, meat only 3 oz	85	65	11	1	2
Canned, solids and liquid, 3 oz	85	45	7	1	2
Crabmeat, canned, 1 cup	135	135	24	3	1
Haddock, breaded, dried, 3 oz	85	140	17	5	5
Ocean perch, breaded, fried, 1 fillet	85	195	16	11	6
Oysters, raw, meat only 1 cup	240	160	20	4	8
Salmon, pink, canned, 3 oz	85	120	17	5	0
Sardines, Atlantic, canned in oil, drained, 3 oz	85	175	20	9	0
Scallops, breaded, fried, 6 scallops	90	175	16	8	9
Shad, baked with butter, 3 oz	85	170	20	10	0
Shrimp:					
Canned meat, 3 oz	85	100	21	1	1
French fried, 3 oz	85	190	17	9	9
Tuna, canned in oil, drained, 3 oz	85	170	24	7	0
Tuna salad, 1 cup	205	350	30	22	7
Meat and meat products:					
Bacon, broiled or fried crisp, 2 slices	15	85	4	8	Trace
Beef, cooked:					
Braised, simmered, pot roasted:					
Lean and fat, 3 oz	85	245	23	16	0
Lean only, 2.5 oz	72	140	22	5	0
Ground beef, broiled:					
Lean with 10% fat, 3 oz	85	185	23	10	0
Lean with 21% fat, 2.9 oz	82	235	20	17	0

TABLE OF MACRO-NUTRIENT VALUES (continued)

	Weight Grams	Energy Calories	Protein Grams	Fat Grams	Carbo-hydrate Grams
Roast, oven cooked:					
Relatively fat, such as rib:					
Lean and fat, 3 oz	85	375	17	33	0
Lean only, 1.8 oz	51	125	14	7	0
Relatively lean, such as					
heel of round:					
Lean and fat, 3 oz	85	165	25	7	0
Lean only, 2.8 oz	78	125	24	3	0
Steak:					
Relatively fat, sirloin,					
broiled:					
Lean and fat, 3 oz	85	330	20	27	0
Lean only, 2.0 oz	56	115	18	4	0
Relatively lean, round,					
braised:					
Lean and fat, 3 oz	85	220	24	13	0
Lean only, 2.4 oz	68	130	21	4	0
Beef, canned:					
Corned beef, 3 oz	85	185	22	10	0
Corned beef hash, 1 cup	220	400	19	25	24
Beef and vegetable stew, 1 cup	245	220	16	11	15
Chili con carne with beans, 1 cup	255	340	19	16	31
Chop suey with beef and pork, 1 cup	250	300	26	17	13
Heart, beef, lean, braised, 3 oz	85	160	27	5	1
Lamb, cooked:					
Chop, rib, broiled:					
Lean and fat, 3.1 oz	89	360	18	32	0
Lean only, 2 oz	57	120	16	6	0
Leg, roasted:					
Lean and fat, 3 oz	85	235	22	16	0
Lean only, 2.5 oz	71	130	20	5	0
Shoulder, roasted:					
Lean and fat, 3 oz	85	285	18	23	0
Lean only, 2.3 oz	64	130	17	6	0
Liver, beef, fried, 3 oz	85	195	22	9	5
Pork, cured, cooked:					
Ham, light cure, lean and fat, 3 oz	85	245	18	19	0
Pork, fresh, cooked:					
Chop, loin, broiled:					
Lean and fat, 2.7 oz	78	305	19	25	0
Lean only, 2 oz	56	150	17	9	0
Roast, oven cooked:					
Lean and fat, 3 oz	85	310	21	24	0
Lean only, 2.4 oz	68	175	20	10	0

TABLE OF MACRO-NUTRIENT VALUES (continued)

	Weight Grams	Energy Calories	Protein Grams	Fat Grams	Carbo-hydrate Grams
Shoulder cut, simmered:					
Lean and fat, 3 oz	85	320	20	26	0
Lean only, 2.2 oz	63	135	18	6	0
Veal, medium fat, cooked, bones removed:					
Cutlet, braised or broiled, 3 oz	85	185	23	9	0
Rib, roasted, 3 oz	85	230	23	14	0
Poultry and poultry products:					
Chicken, cooked:					
Breast, fried, bones removed,					
½ breast, 2.8 oz	79	160	26	5	1
Drumstick, fried, bones					
removed, 1.3 oz	38	90	12	4	Trace
Half broiler, broiled, bones					
removed, 6.2 oz	176	240	42	7	0
Chicken chow mein, canned, 1 cup	250	95	7	Trace	18
Turkey, roasted, flesh without skin:					
Dark meat, piece 2½ by 1⅝					
by ¼ in, 4 pieces	85	175	26	7	0
Light meat, piece 4 by 2 by					
¼ in, 2 pieces	85	150	28	3	0

Fruits and Fruit Products

	Weight Grams	Energy Calories	Protein Grams	Fat Grams	Carbo-hydrate Grams
Apples, raw, unpeeled, without cores:					
Small, 1 apple	138	80	Trace	1	20
Large, 1 apple	212	125	Trace	1	31
Apple juice, 1 cup	248	120	Trace	Trace	30
Applesauce, canned:					
Sweetened, 1 cup	255	230	1	Trace	61
Unsweetened, 1 cup	244	100	Trace	Trace	26
Apricots:					
Raw, without pits, 3 apricots	107	55	1	Trace	14
Dried:					
Uncooked, 1 cup	130	340	7	1	86
Cooked, unsweetened, 1 cup	250	215	4	1	54
Avocados, raw, without skins and seeds:					
California, 1 avocado	216	370	5	37	13
Florida, 1 avocado	304	390	4	33	27
Banana without peel, medium,					
1 banana	119	100	1	Trace	26
Banana flakes, 1 tbsp	6	20	Trace	Trace	5

TABLE OF MACRO-NUTRIENT VALUES (continued)

	Weight Grams	Energy Calories	Protein Grams	Fat Grams	Carbo-hydrate Grams
Blackberries, raw, 1 cup	144	85	2	1	19
Blueberries, raw, 1 cup	145	90	1	1	22
Cantaloupe. See Muskmelons.					
Cherries:					
Sour, red, pitted, canned, water pack, 1 cup	244	105	2	Trace	26
Sweet, raw, without pits and stems, 10 cherries	68	45	1	Trace	12
Cranberries, whole, raw, 1 cup	95	44	Trace	Trace	10
Cranberry juice cocktail, sweetened, 1 cup	253	165	Trace	Trace	42
Cranberry sauce, sweetened, canned, 1 cup	277	405	Trace	1	104
Dates, without pits, 10 dates	80	220	2	Trace	58
Grapefruit, raw, medium:					
Pink or red, ½ grapefruit with peel	241	50	1	Trace	13
White, ½ grapefruit with peel	241	45	1	Trace	12
Grapefruit juice:					
Raw, 1 cup	246	95	1	Trace	23
Canned:					
Unsweetened, 1 cup	247	100	1	Trace	24
Sweetened, 1 cup	250	135	1	Trace	32
Frozen concentrate, unsweetened, diluted by 3 parts water, 1 cup	247	100	1	Trace	24
Grapes, European type, raw:					
Thompson Seedless, 10 grapes	50	35	Trace	Trace	9
Tokay, seeded, 10 grapes	60	40	Trace	Trace	10
Grape juice:					
Canned or bottled, 1 cup	253	165	1	Trace	42
Frozen concentrate, sweetened, diluted with 3 parts water, 1 cup	250	135	1	Trace	33
Lemon, raw, without peel and seeds, 1 lemon	74	20	1	Trace	6
Lemon juice:					
Raw, 1 cup	244	60	1	Trace	20
Bottled, unsweetened, 1 cup	244	55	1	Trace	19
Lemonade concentrate, frozen, diluted, 1 cup	248	105	Trace	Trace	28

TABLE OF MACRO-NUTRIENT VALUES (continued)

	Weight Grams	Energy Calories	Protein Grams	Fat Grams	Carbo-hydrate Grams
Lime juice, raw unsweetened, 1 cup	246	65	1	Trace	22
Muskmelons, raw, with rind, without seeds:					
Cantaloupe, ½ melon	477	80	2	Trace	20
Honeydew, ¹/₁₀ melon	226	50	1	Trace	11
Oranges, raw, medium:					
Whole, 1 orange	131	65	1	Trace	16
Sections, 1 cup	180	90	2	Trace	22
Orange juice:					
Raw, 1 cup	248	110	2	Trace	26
Canned, unsweetened, 1 cup	249	120	2	Trace	28
Frozen concentrate, diluted with					
three parts water, 1 cup	249	120	2	Trace	29
Papayas, raw, ½-in cubes, 1 cup	140	55	1	Trace	14
Peaches:					
Raw:					
Whole, pitted, 1 peach	100	40	1	Trace	10
Sliced, 1 cup	170	65	1	Trace	16
Canned, water pack, 1 cup	244	75	1	Trace	20
Dried:					
Uncooked, 1 cup	160	420	5	1	109
Cooked, unsweetened, 1 cup	250	205	3	1	54
Frozen, sliced, sweetened, 1 cup	250	220	1	Trace	57
Pears, raw, with skin, cored,					
Bartlett, 1 pear	164	100	1	1	25
Pineapple, raw, diced, 1 cup	155	80	1	Trace	21
Pineapple juice, unsweetened,					
canned, 1 cup	250	140	1	Trace	34
Plums, raw, without pits, hybrid					
and Japanese, 1 plum	66	30	Trace	Trace	8
Prunes, dried, with pits:					
Uncooked, 5 large prunes	49	110	1	Trace	29
Cooked, unsweetened, 1 cup	250	255	2	1	67
Prune juice, bottled, 1 cup	256	195	1	Trace	49
Raisins, seedless:					
Cup, not pressed down, 1 cup	145	420	4	Trace	112
Packet, ½ oz or 1½ tbsp	14	40	Trace	Trace	11
Raspberries, red, raw, 1 cup	123	70	1	1	17
Strawberries, raw, capped, 1 cup	149	55	1	1	13

TABLE OF MACRO-NUTRIENT VALUES (continued)

	Weight Grams	Energy Calories	Protein Grams	Fat Grams	Carbo-hydrate Grams
Tangerine, raw, 1 tangerine	86	40	1	Trace	10
Watermelon, raw, 4 by 8 in wedge	926	110	2	1	27

Grain Products

Barley, pearled, uncooked:

Light, 1 cup	200	700	16	2	158
Pot or Scotch, 1 cup	200	696	19	2	154

Breads:

Boston brown bread, 1 slice	45	95	2	1	21
Cracked wheat bread, 1 slice	25	65	2	1	13
French bread, 1 slice	35	100	3	1	19
Italian bread, 1 slice	30	85	3	Trace	17
Raisin bread, 1 slice	25	65	2	1	13
Rye bread, American, 1 slice	25	60	2	Trace	13
Rye bread, Pumpernickel, 1 slice	32	80	3	Trace	17
Whole-wheat bread, 1 slice.....................	25	60	3	1	12

Breakfast cereals:
Hot, cooked:

Corn (hominy) grits, 1 cup.....................	245	125	3	Trace	27
Farina, regular, 1 cup............................	245	103	3	Trace	21
Oatmeal or rolled oats, 1 cup.................	240	130	5	2	23
Wheat, rolled, 1 cup	240	180	5	1	41
Wheat, whole-meal, 1 cup.....................	245	110	4	1	23

Ready-to-eat:

Bran flakes (40% bran), added sugar, 1 cup.....................	35	105	4	1	28
Bran flakes with raisins, sugar, 1 cup.....................	50	145	4	1	40
Corn flakes, plain, added sugar, 1 cup.....................	25	95	2	Trace	21
Corn, puffed, plain, added sugar, 1 cup.....................	20	80	2	1	16
Oats, puffed, added sugar, 1 cup.............................	25	100	3	1	19

Rice, puffed:

Plain, 1 cup	15	60	1	Trace	13
Presweetened, 1 cup........................	28	115	1	0	26
Wheat flakes, added sugar, 1 cup.............................	30	105	3	Trace	24

TABLE OF MACRO-NUTRIENT VALUES (continued)

	Weight Grams	Energy Calories	Protein Grams	Fat Grams	Carbo-hydrate Grams
Wheat, puffed:					
Plain, 1 cup	15	55	2	Trace	12
Presweetened, 1 cup	38	140	3	Trace	33
Wheat, shredded, plain, 1 oblong biscuit or ½ cup spoon-size biscuits	25	90	2	1	20
Wheat germ, without salt and sugar, toasted, 1 tbsp	6	25	2	1	3
Buckwheat flour, sifted:					
Dark, 1 cup	98	326	11	2	70
Light, 1 cup	98	340	6	1	78
Bulgur (parboiled wheat):					
Dry, winter wheat, 1 cup	170	602	19	2	128
Canned, seasoned, 1 cup	135	245	8	4	44
Cornmeal:					
Whole-ground, unbolted, dry, 1 cup	122	435	11	5	90
Bolted, dry, 1 cup	122	440	11	4	91
Corn pone, 9-in diameter by ¾-in thick, baked:					
Whole pone	485	989	21	25	175
Sector, ⅛ of pone	60	122	2	3	21
Crackers:					
Graham, plain, 2 crackers	14	55	1	1	10
Rye, whole-grain, 2 wafers	13	45	2	Trace	10
Muffins, home recipe:					
Blueberry, 1 muffin	40	110	3	4	17
Bran, 1 muffin	40	105	3	4	17
Corn, 1 muffin	40	125	3	4	19
Oatmeal cookies with raisins, 4 cookies	52	235	3	8	38
Pancakes, 4-in diameter:					
Buckwheat, mix, 1 cake	27	55	2	2	6
Plain, home recipe, 1 cake	27	60	2	2	9
Popcorn, popped, plain, 1 cup	6	25	1	Trace	5
Rice:					
Brown, long grain, cooked:					
Served hot, 1 cup	195	232	5	1	49
Served cold, 1 cup	145	173	3	1	37

TABLE OF MACRO-NUTRIENT VALUES (continued)

	Weight Grams	Energy Calories	Protein Grams	Fat Grams	Carbo-hydrate Grams
White, long, grain, cooked:					
Served hot, 1 cup	205	223	4	Trace	49
Served cold, 1 cup	145	158	3	Trace	35
Soybean flour:					
Full fat, stirred, 1 cup	70	295	25	14	21
Low fat, stirred, 1 cup	88	313	38	6	32
Defatted, stirred, 1 cup	100	326	47	1	38
Whole-wheat flour, stirred, 1 cup	120	400	16	2	85
Legumes (Dry), Nuts, Seeds					
Almonds, slivered, 1 cup	115	690	21	62	22
Beans, dry:					
Common varieties, cooked, 1 cup	180	210	14	1	38
Lima, cooked, drained, 1 cup	190	260	16	1	49
Blackeye peas, dry, cooked, 1 cup	250	190	13	1	35
Brazil nuts, shelled, 1 oz	28	185	4	19	3
Cashew nuts, roasted in oil, 1 cup	140	785	24	64	41
Coconut meat, fresh, piece 2 by 2 by ½ in, 1 piece	45	155	2	16	4
Filberts (hazelnuts), chopped, 1 cup	115	730	14	72	19
Lentils, whole, cooked, 1 cup	200	210	16	Trace	39
Peanuts, roasted in shell, shelled:					
Chopped, 1 cup	144	838	37	70	29
Chopped, 1 tbsp	9	52	2	4	2
Peanut butter, 1 tbsp	16	95	4	8	3
Peas, split, dry, cooked, 1 cup	200	230	16	1	42
Pecans, chopped, 1 cup	118	810	11	84	17
Pumpkin seeds, dry, hulled, 1 cup	140	775	41	65	21
Sunflower seeds, dry, hulled, 1 cup	145	810	35	69	29
Walnuts:					
Black, chopped, 1 cup	125	785	26	74	19
English, chopped, 1 cup	120	780	18	77	19
Sugars and Sweets					
Honey, extracted 1 tbsp	21	65	Trace	0	17

TABLE OF MACRO-NUTRIENT VALUES (continued)

	Weight Grams	Energy Calories	Protein Grams	Fat Grams	Carbo-hydrate Grams
Sirups:					
Molasses, cane:					
Light, 1 tbsp	20	50	—	—	13
Blackstrap, 1 tbsp	20	45	—	—	11
Sorghum, tbsp	21	55	—	—	14
Sugars:					
Brown, pressed down, 1 cup	220	820	0	0	212
White, granulated:					
1 cup	200	770	0	0	199
1 tbsp	12	45	0	0	12
1 tsp	4	15	0	0	4

Vegetables and Vegetable Products

	Weight Grams	Energy Calories	Protein Grams	Fat Grams	Carbo-hydrate Grams
Asparagus, green, cut, cooked:					
From raw, 1 cup	145	30	3	Trace	5
From frozen, 1 cup	180	40	6	Trace	6
Beans:					
Lima, frozen, cooked:					
Thick-seeded types, 1 cup	170	170	10	Trace	32
Thin-seeded types, 1 cup	180	210	13	Trace	40
Snap, green, cooked, drained:					
From raw, cuts, 1 cup	125	30	2	Trace	7
From frozen, cuts, 1 cup	135	35	2	Trace	8
Yellow or wax, cooked, drained:					
From raw, cuts, 1 cup	125	30	2	Trace	6
From frozen, cuts, 1 cup	135	35	2	Trace	8
Soybeans, dry, cooked, 1 cup	180	234	19	10	19
Bean sprouts:					
Mung:					
Raw, 1 cup	105	35	4	Trace	7
Cooked, 1 cup	125	35	4	Trace	7
Soybean:					
Raw, 1 cup	105	48	6	1	5
Cooked, 1 cup	125	48	6	1	4
Beets, fresh, cooked, diced, 1 cup	170	55	2	Trace	12
Beet greens, cooked, 1 cup	145	25	2	Trace	5
Blackeye peas, cooked, drained:					
From raw, 1 cup	165	180	13	1	30
From frozen, 1 cup	170	220	15	1	40

TABLE OF MACRO-NUTRIENT VALUES (continued)

	Weight Grams	Energy Calories	Protein Grams	Fat Grams	Carbo-hydrate Grams
Broccoli, cooked, drained:					
From raw, cut, 1 cup	155	40	5	Trace	7
From frozen, chopped, 1 cup	185	50	5	1	9
Brussels sprouts, cooked, drained:					
From raw, 1 cup	155	55	7	1	10
From frozen, 1 cup	155	50	5	Trace	10
Cabbage, common varieties:					
Raw:					
Coarsely shredded, 1 cup	70	15	1	Trace	4
Finely shredded, 1 cup	90	20	1	Trace	5
Cooked, drained, 1 cup	145	30	2	Trace	6
Carrots:					
Raw, without crowns:					
Whole, 1 medium carrot	72	30	1	Trace	7
Grated, 1 cup	110	45	1	Trace	11
Cooked, crosswise cuts, 1 cup	155	50	1	Trace	11
Cauliflower:					
Raw, chopped, 1 cup	115	31	3	Trace	6
Cooked, drained:					
From raw flower buds, 1 cup	125	30	3	Trace	5
From frozen flowerets, 1 cup	180	30	3	Trace	6
Celery, raw:					
1 large outer stalk	40	5	Trace	Trace	2
Pieces, diced, 1 cup	120	20	1	Trace	5
Collards, cooked, drained:					
From raw, leaves, 1 cup	190	65	7	1	10
From frozen, chopped, 1 cup	170	50	5	1	10
Corn, sweet, cooked:					
From raw, 1 medium ear	140	70	2	1	16
From frozen, kernels, 1 cup	165	130	5	1	31
Cucumber slices, 1/8 in thick, with peel, 6 slices from large cucumber or 8 slices from small cucumber	28	5	Trace	Trace	1
Dandelion greens, cooked, 1 cup	105	35	2	1	7
Endive (including escarole), raw, small pieces, 1 cup	50	10	1	Trace	2
Kale, cooked, drained:					
From raw leaves, 1 cup	110	45	5	1	7
From frozen (leaf style), 1 cup	130	40	4	1	7

TABLE OF MACRO-NUTRIENT VALUES (continued)

	Weight Grams	Energy Calories	Protein Grams	Fat Grams	Carbo-hydrate Grams
Lettuce, raw:					
Boston types, 1 outer or 2 inner or 3 heart leaves	15	Trace	Trace	Trace	Trace
Crisphead (Iceberg), chopped, 1 cup	55	5	Trace	Trace	2
Looseleaf (bunching and romaine), chopped, 1 cup	55	10	1	Trace	2
Mushrooms, raw, chopped, 1 cup	70	20	2	Trace	3
Mustard greens, cooked, 1 cup	140	30	3	1	6
Okra pods, cooked, 10 pods	106	30	2	Trace	6
Onions, mature:					
Raw, chopped, 1 cup	170	65	3	Trace	15
Cooked, 1 cup	210	60	3	Trace	14
Parsley, raw, chopped, 1 tbsp	4	Trace	Trace	Trace	Trace
Parsnips, cooked, diced, 1 cup	155	100	2	1	23
Peas, green:					
Canned, drained, 1 cup	170	150	8	1	29
Frozen, cooked, drained, 1 cup	160	110	8	Trace	19
Peppers, sweet:					
Raw, 1 pod	74	15	1	Trace	4
Cooked, boiled, drained, 1 pod	73	15	1	Trace	3
Potatoes, cooked:					
Baked, 1 potato	156	145	4	Trace	33
Boiled, 1 potato	137	105	3	Trace	23
French-fried, strips 2 to 3½ in long, 10 strips	50	135	2	7	18
Potato chips, 1¾ by 2½ in, 10 chips	20	115	1	8	10
Potato salad, made with salad dressing, 1 cup	250	250	7	7	41
Pumpkin, canned, 1 cup	245	80	2	1	19
Radishes, raw, 4 radishes	18	5	Trace	Trace	1
Sauerkraut, canned, 1 cup	235	40	2	Trace	9
Spinach:					
Raw, chopped, 1 cup	55	15	2	Trace	2
Cooked, drained:					
From raw, 1 cup	180	40	5	1	6
From frozen, 1 cup	205	45	6	1	8

TABLE OF MACRO-NUTRIENT VALUES (continued)

	Weight Grams	Energy Calories	Protein Grams	Fat Grams	Carbo-hydrate Grams
Squash, cooked:					
Summer, diced, 1 cup	210	30	2	Trace	7
Winter, baked, mashed, 1 cup	205	130	4	1	32
Sweet potatoes, cooked:					
Baked in skin, 1 potato	114	160	2	1	37
Boiled in skin, 1 potato	151	170	3	1	40
Tomatoes:					
Raw, medium, 1 tomato	135	25	1	Trace	6
Canned, 1 cup	241	50	2	Trace	10
Tomato catsup, 1 tbsp	15	15	Trace	Trace	4
Tomato juice, canned:					
1 cup	243	45	2	Trace	10
1 glass (6 fl oz)	182	35	2	Trace	8
Turnips, cooked, diced, 1 cup	155	35	1	Trace	8
Turnip greens, cooked, drained:					
From raw, 1 cup	145	30	3	Trace	5
From frozen, chopped, 1 cup	165	40	4	Trace	6
Vegetables, mixed, frozen, cooked, 1 cup	182	115	6	1	24
Miscellaneous Items					
Barbecue sauce, 1 cup	250	230	4	17	20
Gelatin, dry, one 7-gram envelope	7	25	6	Trace	0
Gelatin dessert, 1 cup	240	140	4	0	34
Mustard, yellow, 1 tsp	5	5	Trace	Trace	Trace
Olives, pickled, canned:					
Green, 4 medium	16	15	Trace	2	Trace
Ripe, Mission, 3 small	10	15	Trace	2	Trace
Pickles, cucumber:					
Dill, medium, 1 pickle	65	5	Trace	Trace	1
Sweet, small, 1 pickle	15	20	Trace	Trace	5
Relish, sweet, 1 tbsp	15	20	Trace	Trace	5
Soups:					
Canned, prepared with water:					
Bean with pork, 1 cup	250	170	8	6	22

TABLE OF MACRO-NUTRIENT VALUES (continued)

	Weight Grams	Energy Calories	Protein Grams	Fat Grams	Carbo-hydrate Grams
Beef broth, consomme, 1 cup	240	30	5	0	3
Split pea, 1 cup	245	145	9	3	21
Tomato, 1 cup	245	90	2	3	16
Vegetable beef, 1 cup	245	80	5	2	10
Vegetarian, 1 cup	245	80	2	2	13
Dehydrated, ½-in bouillon cube	4	5	1	Trace	Trace
Vinegar, cider, 1 tbsp	15	Trace	Trace	0	1
Yeast, brewer's, dry, 1 tbsp	8	25	3	Trace	3

Note: The listing of foods in my macro-nutrient chart has been abbreviated and simplified for easier reference and easier reading. All unmeasured servings of foods are average or medium in size. If you don't find some of your favorite foods listed, refer to a comparable food for comparison. The chart includes examples of *all* the basic foods, most of which are fresh and prepared in a simple manner. For a complete, alphabetical listing of all types of foods prepared in a variety of ways and measured in specific amounts, see *Nutritive Value of American Foods in Common Units,* Agriculture Handbook No. 456, available from the Superintendent of Documents, U.S. Government Printing Office, Washington, D.C. 20402.

MACRO-NUTRIENT FOOD SOURCES OF
IMPORTANT MICRO-NUTRIENTS

In a balanced diet of macro-nutrient foods, there is considerable overlapping of food sources of essential nutrients. Some foods are more concentrated than others in certain nutrients, however. If you eat foods from all the basic food groups each day, you'll automatically include the macro-nutrient foods that supply the essential micro-nutrients. But when you want to enrich your diet with a particular micro-nutrient, you should increase your intake of selected foods. Following is a list of some important micro-nutrient food sources.

Vitamins

Vitamin A: Yellow fruits and vegetables, such as peaches, carrots, and sweet potatoes; dried fruits, such as apricots; whole dairy products, especially milk, cheese, and butter; beef liver, egg yolk; enriched margarine.

Vitamin B complex: Meats, whole-grain products, poultry, fish, eggs, brewer's yeast, wheat germ, liver, legumes, milk. (Vitamin B$_{12}$ is found only in foods of animal origin.)

Vitamin C: Citrus fruits, tomatoes, strawberries, bean sprouts, broccoli, cabbage, cauliflower.

Vitamin D: Enriched milk, egg yolk, saltwater fish, liver, sunflower seeds.

Vitamin E: Vegetable oils, margarine, whole-grain breads and cereals, peanuts, wheat germ, wheat germ oil.

Folic acid: Liver, dark green vegetables, dry beans, peanuts, wheat germ.

Minerals

Calcium: Milk, cheese, yogurt, dark green leafy vegetables, whole-grain breads, sardines and salmon canned with bones.

Iron: Red meats, liver, dried fruits, whole-grain products, dark green leafy vegetables, legumes.

Iodine: Seafood, iodized salt, kelp.

Zinc: Shellfish (especially oysters), meat, cheese, whole-grain cereals, dry beans, nuts

Potassium: Meats, cereals, fruits, fruit juices, vegetables.

Index

A

A, vitamin, 230
Accidents, 167
Additives, 64, 157
Alcohol, 167
Alkalizers, 134
Allergy, gluten, 175–176
Amino acids, 21, 22
Anemia, 67, 87
Appearance, 184, 196–197
Appestat, 185
Appetite, 185–186
Arteriosclerosis, 167
Arthritis:
  fight, 179–180
  gouty, 17, 67, 178–179
  osteo, 180
  rheumatoid, 180
Artificial sweetners, 31
Atherosclerosis, 23, 33
Attractiveness, 196

B

Basal metabolic rate, 54
Basic foods, 29–30
Basketball, calories, 187
B complex vitamins, 230
Beans, 29, 30
Bedtime snack, 205, 207, 208, 209, 210,
  212
Beef, 22

Behavior modification:
  coffee breaks, 194–195
  junk food in home, 193–194
  no business meals, 192
  no meals at parties, 192–193
  slow eating, 191
  small plates, 192
  thorough chewing, 191
  using food as tranquilizer, 193
  when you eat, 190–191
  where you eat, 190–191
Benefits, 202–204
Betaine hydrochloride, 181
Beverages, 34
Bicycling, calories, 187
Blood fat, 169
Blood pressure, 17–18, 67
Blood sugar, 35
Blood vessel disease, 169
Blood vessels, 23
Body:
  proportions, 184
  supplements, 181 (*see also* Supple-
    ments)
Boredom, 193
Bowling, calories, 187
Bran:
  fiber, 117–118, 129–130, 131–132 (*see*
    also Fiber)
  miller's 33, 89, 129
  nibbling, 145–148 (*see also* Nibbling)
Bran flakes, 127
Bread:
  fiber, 126
  whole-grain, 29, 30, 33

Breakfast, 35, 47, 205, 206, 207, 209, 210, 211
Bronchopulmonic diseases, 167
Brownies, bran, 131–132
Bulgur, 127
Business meals, 192
Butter, 29
Butterfat, 26

C

C, vitamin, 230
Cake, carob carrot brand, 132
Calcium, 162, 230
Calories:
  amount to consume, 25–26
  anorexia nervosa, 69
  average person, 61
  basic energy nutrients, 59
  basic food groups, 60
  best weight, 68–69
  burn fat by eating, 66–67
  carbohydrate high, 59–60
  diet balanced for lifetime, 50–51
  diet results vary, 61–63
  energy nutrients, 40–42, 46
  exercise, 51–52, 58–59, 186–187 (*see also* Exercise)
  fasting, 66–68
  fat low, 59–60
  figure requirement, 56–59
  gram figures, 59
  keep stomach full, 50–51
  low-carbohydrate diets, 68
  maintenance diet, 62
  meat, 48, 50
  monitor your weight, 62
  natural carbohydrates, 22
  nutritious vs. empty, 55
  1,200 diet, 40, 44–45, 204–205, 209–210
  1,500 + diet, 206–207, 210
  2,000 diet, 40–42
  2,500 + diet, 207–208, 211–212
  output, 55
  quick review, 59
  refined-carbohydrate, 56
  retention of water, 60–61
  salt intake, 63–64
  tailor intake, 54

Calories (*cont'd*)
  three-meal menu, 47–48
  water, 64–66
  weight charts, 57
  weight loss, 57–59, 60–61
  you are unique, 48–49
Cancer:
  balanced diet, 174
  colon, 116
  dietary fat, 17, 33
  nutritional deficiencies, 173–174
Canned foods, 31
Carbohydrates:
  cellulose, 24
  Chinese people, 25
  complex, 24–25, 26
  diabetics, 23
  early 1900's, 22
  fiber, 24–25
  low in calories, 22–23
  minimum dietary requirements, 22
  natural, 18, 22, 23, 24, 25, 27
  prevent disease, 23–24
  prevent heart disease, 23
  principal body fuel, 23
  refined, 18, 22, 23, 24, 56
  Seventh Day Adventists, 25
Cardiovascular disease, 169
Carob carrot bran cake, 132
Catsup, 31
Celebrities, 154–156
Celiac disease, 176
Cellulose, 24, 118, 147
Central nervous system, 167
Cereals, 32, 33, 127
Charts, weight, 57
Chewing food, 191
Children, milk and eggs, 26
Chinese people, 25
Chinese restaurants, 157
Cholesterol, 23, 25, 26, 91, 118, 169, 170–172
Chromium deficiency, 174
Cigarettes, 167
Cirrhosis of liver, 167
Coffee breaks, 194–195
Cola, 31
Colon:
  bran, 148
  cancer, 116, 173
  clean, 177

Constipation, 147, 177
Corn pone, 126–127
Cottage cheese, 33
Cracked wheat, 127
Crude fiber, 118

D

D, vitamin, 230
Dairy products, 26, 77, 215–216
Dancing, calories, 187
Death, causes, 167
Dehydration, 21
Depression, 193
Desserts, 131, 156
Diabetes mellitus, 167, 174–175
Diabetics, 23, 144
Diarrhea:
  celiac disease, 176
  diverticulitis, 177
Diet:
  "bran," 118
  maintenance, 39
  1,200 calorie, 40, 44–45, 204–205,
    209–210
  1,500 + calories, 206–207, 210
  2,000 calorie, 40–42
  2,500 + calories, 207–208, 211–212
  results vary, 61–63
  vegetarian, 105–108
Dietary fiber, 118
Dietary Goals for the United States, 23,
  24, 25–27
Diet plan, 35–36
Diet revolution, 20–22
Dinner, 36, 47, 205, 206, 208, 209, 210,
  212
Dip, yogurt, 142
Disease, prevent, 23–24, 33
Diverticulitis, 116, 176–177
Dressing, Italian, 143
Drinking alcohol, 167
Drinks:
  enrich, 112–113
  formula, 110–111
  meal-substitute, 109–113
  only one meal, 110

E

E, vitamin, 230

Eating:
  business meals, 192
  chewing, 191
  coffee breaks, 194–195
  emotions, 193
  junk food, 193–194
  parties, 192–193
  slowly, 191
  small plates, 192
  when, 190–191
  where, 190–191
Eggs, 26, 29, 33, 80–81, 216
Elderly, 26
Emotions, 193
Energy nutrients:
  calculate percentages, 46
  1,200 calorie diet, 40
  2,000 calorie diet, 40–42
Exercise:
  appestat, 185
  calories burned, 54–55, 58–59, 186–187
  combined with diet, 51–52, 189
  get most for effort, 186
  governs appetite, 185–186
  lack, disease, 167
  maintenance program, 184–189
  research, 185
  strengthen heart, 172
  walking, 187–188

F

Fast-food, 154
Fasting:
  anemia, 67
  burn more fat by eating, 66
  carbohydrate, 66
  day or two, 66
  fall in blood pressure, 67
  fatigue, 67
  glucose, 66
  glycogen, 66
  gouty arthritis, 67
  hair loss, 66
  headache, 67
  heart rate, 66
  ketones, 66
  loss of minerals, 66
  low-carbohydrate diets, 68
  metabolic functions, 66

Fasting *(cont'd)*
  muscle protein, 67, 68, 69
  nausea, 67
  nutritional deficiencies, 66
  periodically, 67
  prolonged, 66
  starvation, 66
  traveling, 158–159
Fasting blood sugar, 145
Fatigue, 67
Fat:
  blood, 169
  burned, 92
  cooking with, 33
  hidden, 151
  manipulate, 153–154
  minimum, 90–93
  nutrient values, 216–217
  polyunsaturated, 26
  toxic ketones, 17
  trans-fat, 92
  visible, 92–93, 151, 152
Fermented milk product, 75
Fiber:
  add to foods, 128–129
  amount needed, 118–119
  balanced diet, 117, 118
  best sources, 33, 120–121
  bran, 117–118, 129–130
  bran brownies, 131–132
  bran muffins, 130
  carob carrot bran cake, 132
  cellulose, 117
  cereals, 127
  colon cancer, 116
  complex carbohydrates, 24
  conserve in vegetables, 128
  cooking grains, 117
  corn pone, 126–127
  crude, 118
  desserts, 131
  dietary, 118
  diverticulitis, 116, 176–177
  dried beans, 121
  food servings, 125
  grams, 122–125
  hardened arteries, 116
  hemorrhoids, 116
  increase your intake, 117
  irregularity, 130
  make granola, 127–128

Fiber *(cont'd)*
  mineral deficiency, 117
  moisturize colon, 121
  nuts, 121
  overweight, 130
  peas, 121
  phytates, 117
  popular foods, 119–120
  prevents diseases, 116
  raw berries, 120
  raw fruits, 120
  reduce blood cholesterol, 118
  seeds, 121
  selecting and preparing, 125
  types, 117–118
  vegetable, 118
  water-holding, 118
Fish:
  basic food, 29, 30, 33
  cholesterol, 99
  grams of fat, 100
  iodine, 99
  low-fat protein, 99
  low in sodium, 99
  nutrient values, 27
  remove skin, 100
  shellfish, 99, 100
Flour, white, 31, 32, 143
Folic acid, 230
Foods:
  adding fiber, 128–129
  basic, 29–30, 31–35, 60
  preparation, 73
  problems, 73–74
  restaurants *(see* Restaurant food)
Fried food, 154, 155
Fruits, 29, 30, 33, 35, 81–87, 219–222
Frustration, 193

G

Glucose, 23, 24, 66, 143, 193
Glucose tolerance test, 144
Gluten allergy, 175–176
Glycogen, 66, 143
Golf, calories, 187
Gouty arthritis, 17, 67, 178–179
Grains, 24, 26, 29, 222–224
Granola, 127–128
Grape Nuts, 127
Grocery store, 156, 158–159

H

Hair loss, 66
Handball, calories, 187
Hardened arteries, 116
Headaches, 67
Heart disease:
  cause of death, 167
  cholesterol, 170–172
    control, 170
    good guys, 171–172
    natural carbohydrates, 171
    saturated fat, 170–171
  dietary fat, 17, 23
  exercise, 172
Heart rate, 66
Hemorrhoids, 116
Heredity, 167
High-density lipoproteins, 172
High-fat diet, 20–21
Hyperlipidema, 23
Hypoglycemia:
  automatic correction, 145–146
  diagnosis, 144–145
  fasting blood sugar, 145
  functional, 145
  glucose, 143
  glucose tolerance, test, 144
  glycogen and fat, 143
  high-protein snacks, 145, 146
  natural carbohydrates, 144
  obesity, 144
  organic, 145
  pancreas, 143
  refined carbohydrates, 143
  self-treatment, 145
  sugar, 143
  symptoms, 143
  white flour, 143

I

Infancy, diseases, 167
Influenza, 167
Insulin, 23
Intestinal bacteria, 147
Iodine, sources, 230
Iron:
  foods, 163–164, 230
  toxic, 163

Irregularity, 130
Italian dressing, 143

J

Jogging, calories, 187
Junk food, 193–194

K

Ketones, 17, 21, 66
Kidneys:
  frequent urination, 21
  overworked, 17
Kidney stones, 17

L

Labels, 32
Lacto-ovo-vegetarian diet, 105, 179
Lactose, intolerance, 75
Life style, 195
Linoleic acid, 91
Liquid protein diet, 21
Liver, cirrhosis, 167
Loneliness, 193
Low blood sugar, 136, 143–145 (*see also* Hypoglycemia)
Low carbohydrate diets, 17
Low-density lipoproteins, 172
Low-fat milk, 74–75
Lunch, 36, 47, 205, 206, 207, 209, 210, 211
Lunch box:
  avoid lunch meats, 157
  basic food groups, 157
  grocery store, 156, 158–159
  no mayonnaise, 157
  not overeating, 158
  snack on job, 158

M

Magnesium, 65
Maintenance:
  appestat, 185
  appetite, 185–186

Maintenance *(cont'd)*
  calories burned, 186–187
  chew thoroughly, 191
  coffee breaks, 194–195
  diet and exercise, 189
  eat slowly, 191
  exercise, 184–189
  food as tranquilizer, 193
  happiness regained, 197
  junk food, 193–194
  modify behavior, 189–195
  no business meals, 192
  no meals at parties, 192–193
  nutrition, 195–196
  physical attractiveness, 196
  regular schedule, 195
  sedentary people, 185
  sex and appearance, 196–198
  small glasses, 192
  small plates, 192
  take charge, 195–197
  walking, 187–188
  when you eat, 190–191
  where you eat, 191–197
  you are unique, 184
Malignant neoplasms, 167
Margarine, 29, 91–92
Meats:
  cheaper, leaner, 77–78
  fat-rich, 22, 29
  lean, 29, 30, 33
  lunch, 157
  nutrient values, 217–219
  nutrients, 77–81
  selecting, 81
  slimming diet, 48
  substitutes, 78–81, 96–99
Men, weight chart, 57
Menus:
  basic food groups, 201
  benefits of diet, 202–204
  body maintenance, 207
  calorie requirement, 200–201
  calories essential, 208
  common sense, 212
  flexible, 212
  food groups, 212
  food selections, 201
  imagination, 212
  nutrient values, 202
  1,200 + calories, 47, 204–205, 209–210

Menus *(cont'd)*
  1,500 + calories, 206–207, 210
  2,500 + calories, 207–208, 211–212
  pick suitable plan, 200
  rapid weight-loss, 204
  salad as meal, 212
  sample ones for everyone, 208–212
  simply guides, 212
  slower weight loss, 206–207
  smaller portions, 212
  snacks, 212
  use samples, 204
  variety of foods, 212
  waste and expense, 213
Metabolic functions, 66
Milk:
  cow's, 26, 29, 30, 74–77
  soy, 99
Miller's bran, 33, 89, 129
Minerals, food sources, 230
Modification of behavior, 189–195 (*see also* Behavior modification)
Monosodium glutamate, 64, 157
Muffins, bran, 130
Muscle protein, 67, 68, 69
Muscles, develop, 184

N

Nausea, 67
Neoplasms, malignant, 167
Nervousness, 193
Nervous system, 167
New England Journal of Medicine, 17
Nibbling:
  bran, 145–148
    adverse effects, 148
    between meals, 147
    cellulose, 147
    drink water, 148
    how much, 147–148
    intestinal bacteria, 147
    intestinal gas, 148
    mineral-blocking, 147
    not at mealtime, 147
    prevent constipation, 147
    simple snacks, 148
    skim milk, 148
    "stomach filler," 146
    stools, 148

Nibbling *(cont'd)*
    too much, 148
    wheat germ, 148
    divide food intake, 135
    low blood sugar, 136, 143–145 *(see also*
        Hypoglycemia)
    natural carbohydrates, 135
    no processed foods, 135
    pick best method, 137
    popcorn, 142
    raw vegetables, 136, 141–143
      chew, 142
      dressing, recipe, 143
      liquefy, 142
      salad, 142–143
      suggestions, 141–142
      use dip, 141, 142
      yogurt dip, 142
    six times daily, 136, 138–141
      complete protein, 139
      1,200 calories, 139–140
      quick review, 139
      your needs, 138
    soybeans, toasted, 136
    weight goal, 135
Nutrient values:
  food sources, 229–230
  minerals, 230
  results of dieting, 214–215
  table, 215–229
    dairy products, 215–216
    eggs, 216
    fats and oils, 216–217
    fish and shellfish, 217
    fruit, 219–222
    grain, 222–224
    legumes, nuts, seeds, 224–225
    meat, 217–219
    miscellaneous items, 228–229
    poultry, 219
    vegetables, 225–228
  vitamins, 230
Nutrients:
  eggs, 80–81
  fats and oils, 90–93
    burned, 92
    cold-pressed, 91
    cooking, 91
    linoleic acid, 91
    margarine, 91–92
    trans-fat, 92

Nutrients *(cont'd)*
    visible fat, 92–93
  food preparation, 73
  food problems, 73–74
  fresh foods, 72
  liquid protein diet, 21
  meat, 77–81
    cheaper, leaner, 77–78
    selection, 81
    substitutes, 78–81
  milk group, 74–77
    calcium, 76
    cutting the fat, 74–75
    fermented, 75–76
    lactose intolerance, 75
    synthetics, 77
    vitamin B$_{12}$, 76
    yogurt, 75, 76
  overlap sources, 86–87
  peanut butter, 79–80, 92
  requirements, 22
  soybeans, 78–79
  variety of foods, 29
  vegetables and fruits, 81–87
    cook fresh, 86
    cooking, 83–84
    peelings, 85–86
    steam, 84
    vitamin A, 82–83, 84–85
    vitamin C, 82–83, 84
    water-rich, 85
  wheat, 87–88, 89–90
    allergy, 90
    no. 1 grain, 87–88
    warning, 89–90
  whole-grains, 87–90
Nutritional deficiencies, 66

O

Oats, 127
Oil:
  not use in cooking, 33
  nutrient values, 216–217
  vegetable, 25, 29, 34
1,200 calorie diet, 40, 44–45, 47, 204–205,
    209–210
1,500 calorie diet, 206–207, 210
Osteoarthritis, 180
Overweight, 130
Oysters, 33

P

Pancreas, 23–24, 143
Parties, 192–193
Peanut butter, 32, 79–80
Peas, 29, 30
Pectin, 118
Physical appearance, 184, 196–197
Phytic acid, 89
Pneumonia, 167
Polyunsaturated fats, 26
Popcorn, 142
Pork, 22
Potassium, 21, 64, 230
Potatoes, 24
Poultry, 29, 30, 33, 219
Preservatives, 64, 157
Processed foods, 31, 32, 64, 135
Proportions, body, 184
Protein:
    fish, 99–100
    gouty arthritis, 17
    kidney stones, 17
    liquid, 21
    low-calorie, 17, 18
    meal-substitute drinks, 109–113
    salads, 108–109
    snacks, 145, 146
    soybeans, 96–99 (*see also* Soybeans)
    vegetarianism, 105–108
    whole-grain bread, 102–104
    yogurt, 101–102
Pulse rate, 169
Purines, 17, 178, 179

R

Raw vegetables, 136, 141–143
Recipes:
    bran brownies, 131–132
    bran muffins, 130
    carob carrot bran cake, 132
    corn pone, 126–127
    energy drinks, 111
    granola, 127–128
    Italian dressing, 143
    whole-wheat bread, 104
    yogurt dip, 142
Refined carbohydrates, 18, 22, 23, 24, 56,
    143

Restaurant food:
    casseroles, 151
    celebrities, 154–156
    Chinese food, 157
    complete meal, 151–152
    desserts, 156
    fancy dishes, 151
    fast-food, 154, 155
    fattening, 155
    fried foods, 154, 155
    hidden fat, 151
    low in nutrients, 150–151
    manipulate fat, 153–154
    natural carbohydrates, 152, 153
    new or unfamiliar foods, 154–155
    oils, 151
    overcooked vegetable, 150, 151
    refined carbohydrates, 152, 153
    sample low-fat meal, 154
    seasoning, 151
    selecting, 151–154
    take own lunch, 155–156
    visible fat, 151, 152
Results:
    average, 61
    report, 214
    vary, 61–63
Rheumatoid arthritis, 180

S

Safflower oil, 34, 91
Salad:
    between-meal, 142
    complete meal, 108–109
    dark leaves, 108
    enrich, 108–109
    Italian dressing, 143
    raw, 33, 34, 108
Salt, 26, 27, 63–64
Saturated fats, 26
Sauces, 151, 155
Schedule, regular, 195
Sedentary people, 185
Seven basic food groups, 29–30, 60
Seventh Day Adventists, 23, 25
Sex, 196–197
Shredded wheat, 127
Skating, calories, 187
Skiing, calories, 187

Skim milk, 29, 30, 34, 74–75, 148
Slimming program:
　diet balanced for lifetime, 50–51
　energy-nutrient percentages, 46
　exercising, 51–52
　long-range, 42–44
　meat, 48
　1,200 calorie, 40, 44–45
　protein intake, 39
　sample menu, 47
　2,000 calorie, 40–42
　you are unique, 48–49
Smoking, 167
Snacks (*see* Nibbling)
Sodium:
　limit intake, 26, 63–64
　loss, 17, 18
Sodium nitrate, 64, 157
Softball, calories, 187
Soft drinks, 31
Soybeans:
　cooking, 96–97
　discard cooking water, 97
　dry, 96, 97
　field, 96
　green, 96
　nearly equal to meat, 78–79
　soy milk, 99
　sprouts, 97–98
　　grow, 97–98
　　how to cook, 98
　toasted, 136
　vegetable, 96
　warning, 96
Sprouts, soy, 97–98
Starvation, 66
Stir frying, 25
Stools:
　bran, 148
　celiac disease, 176
Stress, 167
Sugar:
　canned foods, 31
　catsup, 31
　do not use, 31
　low blood sugar, 143
　"naturally occurring," 26
　refined and processed, 26, 27
Sunflower oils, 91
Supplements:
　calcium, 162

Supplements (*cont'd*)
　iron, 163–164
　vitamins, 159–162, 164–165
　wisdom of body, 181
Sweeteners, 31
Sweets, craving, 35, 136
Swimming, calories, 187
Sympathetic nervous system, 17

T

Tennis, calories, 187
Tranquilizer, food, 193
Traveling, 158–159
Triglycerides, 25, 169
2,000 calorie diet, 40–42
2,500 + calorie diet, 207–208, 211–212

U

Unleavened bread, 89
Uric acid, 17, 21, 178

V

Vascular lesions, 167
Veal, 33
Vegetable oil, 25, 29, 34, 91
Vegetable juices, 34
Vegetables, 29, 30, 33, 81, 82–87, 128, 136, 141–143, 225–228 (*see also* Nibbling)
Vegetarian diet:
　balancing, 105–106
　food plan, 106–107
　fruits and vegetables, 106
　milk or milk products, 106
　nonfattening, 105
　planning meals, 107–108
　protein foods, 106
　Seventh Day Adventists, 25
　whole grains, 106
Vitamins:
　food sources, 230
　larger doses, 160–162, 164
　needs differ, 164
　special reasons, 164–165
　water-soluble, 159–160

W

Walking, calories, 187–188
Water:
  drink plenty, 63
  following bran, 148
  mineral, 65
  natural carbohydrates, 65
  retention, 60–61
  your body, 65–66
Weighing, 60–61
Weight charts, 57
Wheat, 87–88, 89–90
Wheat germ, 148
White flour, 31, 32, 143
Whole-grain breads:
  basic foods, 29, 30, 33
  fiber, 104
  not fattening, 103–104
  recipe, 104
  refrigerate, 103
  restaurants, 102
  weight reduction, 103
Whole-grain flour, 32
Whole grains, 24, 26, 29, 33, 87–90,
    222–224
Whole milk, 74, 75

Women:
  premenstrual, 26
  weight chart, 57

Y

Yogurt:
  commercial maker, 102
  commercial manufacturers, 101
  dip, 142
  eat by itself, 101
  flavor, 102
  fresh, 101
  lactic acid, 101
  live bacteria, 101
  made from skim milk, 33, 76
  making, 102
  snacks, 136
  unique properties, 101–102

Z

Zinc:
  deficiency, 174–175
  sources, 230